Promoting Young People's through Empowerment an(

The terms 'wellbeing', 'empowerment' and 'agency' are common parlance in policy and practice with children, young people and families (CYPF), yet are often misused or not fully understood. Further, there is a disconnect between these abstract concepts and tangible practice with CYPF.

This book bridges the theory-practice divide, offering a clear and definitive guide to concepts and practical ways to develop CYPF wellbeing. It examines the concept of wellbeing and its intrinsic relationship to social justice both theoretically and through case study material, and locates these practices within critical pedagogy. The book highlights a range of practice with CYPF of various ages, in formal and non-formal learning situations, engaged in a range of different programmes including learning, reduction from offending, social action and tackling targeted needs. Each chapter highlights relevant policy, research and practice examples to ensure that the book is relevant to a variety of readers.

This book will benefit students and practitioners who work with young people to realise wellbeing and to embed critical pedagogy in their practice. It also provides a frame of reference to critically engage in policy analysis and is essential reading for social workers, teachers, police support officers and anyone working to support CYPF to become empowered.

Lucy Maynard is Head of Research at the Brathay Trust. Lucy is a participatory action researcher, working within practice with children, young people and families, to better understand the process of empowerment and agency in wellbeing. This is in order to develop practice and inform the sector and policy.

Kaz Stuart is Principal Lecturer at the University of Cumbria, UK. Kaz manages a range of degree programmes that support practitioners who will work with CYPF. Kaz is an active researcher driven by a passion for wellbeing and social justice, whether that be for CYPF, practitioners or lecturers.

Promoting Young People's Wellbeing through Empowerment and Agency

A Critical Framework for Practice

Lucy Maynard and Kaz Stuart

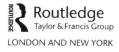
Routledge
Taylor & Francis Group

LONDON AND NEW YORK

First published 2018
by Routledge
2 Park Square, Milton Park, Abingdon, Oxon OX14 4RN

and by Routledge
711 Third Avenue, New York, NY 10017

Routledge is an imprint of the Taylor & Francis Group, an informa business

British Library Cataloguing in Publication Data
A catalogue record for this book is available from the British Library

Library of Congress Cataloging in Publication Data
Names: Maynard, Lucy, author. | Stuart, Kaz, author.
Title: Promoting young people's wellbeing through empowerment and
agency : a critical framework for practice / Lucy Maynard and
Karen Stuart.
Description: Abingdon, Oxon ; New York, NY : Routledge, 2017. | Includes
bibliographical references and index.
Identifiers: LCCN 2017005826 | ISBN 9781138937185 (hardback) |
ISBN 9781138937192 (pbk.) | ISBN 9781315676418 (ebook)
Subjects: LCSH: Social work with youth. | Youth--Social conditions. |
Youth--Services for. | Well-being. | Youth development.
Classification: LCC HV1421 .M37 2017 | DDC 362.7--dc23
LC record available at https://lccn.loc.gov/2017005826

ISBN: 978-1-138-93718-5 (hbk)
ISBN: 978-1-138-93719-2 (pbk)
ISBN: 978-1-315-67641-8 (ebk)

Typeset in Times New Roman
by Taylor & Francis Books

We wish to dedicate this book to the children, young people, families and practitioners who have inspired us.

Contents

viii   *Contents*

Illustrations

Boxes

List of cases / vignettes

Acknowledgements

We would like to extend our thanks to all the people and practitioners that have supported the development of this book. This has been through patient support of our joys and frustrations, through allowing us access to your worlds, and for allowing us to publish your narratives and experiences. In particular, thanks needs to go to:

- Brathay Trust
- Eikon
- Aaron
- Gemma
- The Aspiring Leaders
- Charlotte Hardacre
- Emma Perris and The Foyer Federation
- Jane Robinson.

Introduction

We hear the term 'wellbeing' on a daily basis, in a variety of contexts and through a variety of media. Managers, leaders, organisations, services, practitioners and policy makers are increasingly concerned about wellbeing. But why is this? Has people's wellbeing been decreasing, or are we simply more aware of it as a concept and our ability to influence it? There is certainly an argument that people are no longer able or happy to just 'survive'. The work of Positive Psychology has advocated the position of thriving and not simply surviving. Only in recent history in the Western world do we have the time to consider how we experience wellbeing as our survival is now taken for granted. Wellbeing is gradually being seen as a human right rather than a privilege, and as such it is attracting interest from a variety of stakeholders.

And what of the relationship of wellbeing to mental health? Is wellbeing being used as a proxy-measure of mental health? Further, is it a personal construct or something to be considered from a social perspective? These fundamental questions warrant further exploration.

Our particular area of interest in this book is work with children, young people and families (CYPF). Their 'wellbeing' received heightened attention in the UK with the Every Child Matters (DfES, 2004) and Youth Matters (DfES, 2005) agendas. These strengthened the requirement of agencies to work together to ensure children and young people all attained a range of holistic outcomes that could broadly be said to encapsulate wellbeing. Since that time, wellbeing has again been positioned within health in the UK rather than all services for children and young people, as in the *Improving Young People's Health and Wellbeing Framework* (Public Health England, 2015).

So, is wellbeing just the buzzword of the moment, or is it a helpful construct that encapsulates the work we have always done to support CYPF to learn and develop? There is no doubt that the amount of time committed to supporting wellbeing has collectively increased. However, we would like to look at wellbeing through a slightly different lens; one that fits our particular practice with CYPF.

We implicitly know we are working to develop CYPF wellbeing through our work, but how do we do this? This book draws out a variety of practices; making it something explicit. The book summarises a particular approach to developing wellbeing that is of practical use. This approach can be used to frame practice in order to help plan and deliver, as well as critique and evaluate.

What is wellbeing?

Wellbeing has a broad definition and has been considered from multiple perspectives that encompass many aspects of CYPF development. Below we detail some of these critical perspectives to help understand what wellbeing is and to set the context before considering how we facilitate the development of wellbeing.

Perhaps fundamentally we need a definition as a basis for this critical exploration. We subscribe to the notion that wellbeing is about how one feels about one's self and situation and therefore how we feel able to act in the world based on this feeling. Aked *et al.* (2008) summarise this with their stance that,

> ... feelings of happiness, contentment, enjoyment, curiosity and engage-ment, to be characteristic of someone who has a positive experience of their life. Equally important for well-being is our functioning in the world (pp. 1–2)

Therefore, as a foundational reference point, in the multi-dimensional context of wellbeing, we define wellbeing to be *feeling good and functioning well*.

People's functional ability can be understood across a range of domains, including physical, psychological, emotional, intellectual and spiritual. This view is supported by a range of authors (Henderson *et al.*, 2007; Margo and Sodha, 2007: 8; Aked et al., 2008: 1–2). This is not to say that there is consensus on the definition of wellbeing – quite the opposite is true.

We deliberately focus on the functional aspects of wellbeing because it is holistic. We believe that functioning well comes from a delicate balance of all types of wellbeing in interaction with the places and societies in which we live. It is through this lens that we interrogate the concepts of social justice, agency and empowerment.

Wellbeing is considered in different ways by different people and as such can be confusing. There are, however, some key differences in the distinguishing factors of wellbeing.

Objective and subjective wellbeing

A common distinction to consider is one of objectivity and subjectivity. This is particularly debated when people consider the measurement of wellbeing, or changes in wellbeing.

For some, wellbeing is something that is *objective* and measurable. This means that it can be seen and counted, for example, by measuring levels of cortisol to monitor stress (European Society of Endocrinology, 2011). From this objective perspective, indicators of wellbeing that are precisely measurable include: income, poverty, birth weight, percentiles of worklessness, percentiles of academic achievement, percentiles of substance abuse and percentiles of teenage pregnancy.

Other authors define wellbeing as **subjective** and a feeling that can only be self-assessed and reported (Layard, 2002). Components of subjective wellbeing include: positive self-regard, perception of health, enjoyment of life, sense of vitality, levels of resilience, feelings of safety, emotional wellbeing, sense of trust and belonging. It is obvious that these are not measurable with any external scientific tool, they are internal feelings.

Critiques of this subjectivity, focus on these issues of measurement. They suggest that because it is personal, it is not comparable, and therefore measurement and understanding levels of wellbeing are redundant. Supporters of the subjective approach counter that personal feelings and attitudes are measurable, but with rich qualitative narrative tools, rather than statistical quantitative tools (White *et al.*, 2012).

A further distinction can be made between the subjective aspects of wellbeing, distinguishing those that are **emotional** and **psychological**. Emotions and life satisfaction are known as **hedonic** components, and the psychological components are known as **eudaimonic** aspects of wellbeing. The eudaimonic aspects include self-acceptance, positive relationships, autonomy, purpose in life and personal growth. When these are in place, people are said to experience positive wellbeing (The Children's Society, 2013).

From the discussion so far, we can create a conceptual continuum of wellbeing. At one end is the objective conceptualisation of wellbeing and at the other is the subjective conceptualisation of wellbeing. In the middle is a hybrid perspective where wellbeing is perceived to comprise both objective and subjective components. This is shown in Table I.1 below.

Personal and social wellbeing

Another common distinction is made between **personal** and **social** wellbeing.

Personal wellbeing is concerned with an individual's experiences of their emotions, satisfaction, vitality, resilience and self-esteem and sense of positive functioning in the world. Both subjective and objective views of personal wellbeing can be made. Personal subjective wellbeing could focus on feelings, whilst objective personal wellbeing could focus on blood pressure.

Table I.1 The conceptual continuum of wellbeing

Objective perspective of wellbeing	Objective and subjective view of wellbeing	Subjective view of wellbeing (hedonic and eudaimonic)
Precisely measurable with scientific tools	Measured with a combination of tools	Measured with qualitative social science tools

In contrast, social wellbeing is concerned with people's experiences of supportive relationships and sense of trust and belonging with others, as well as within the world (Michaelson *et al.*, 2009:4), and therefore, we would add, their relative functioning in the world. A social subjective perspective could be interested in perceptions of community safety, whilst a social objective stance would be interested in absolute levels of crime within that community.

When we layer the personal social spectrum over the objective subjective spectrum we end up with a matrix of six perspectives of wellbeing. These are shown in Table I.2 below.

Within this book we are writing from the middle perspective. We believe that objective and subjective measures of wellbeing are equally important and that the personal has to be viewed alongside the social as we live within societies. A good example of this is reported in *The Good Childhood Report* (The Children's Society, 2013) where young people's self-reported low satisfaction with life increased with disadvantages such as poverty. This shows that subjective personal wellbeing (life satisfaction) is intrinsically linked to objective personal and social wellbeing (personal wealth and socio-economic deprivation).

Many countries have national measures of personal objective wellbeing. Some examples from the UK are listed below:

- 2.3 million children live in relative low income, and 2.6 million under the absolute low income measure (Department for Work and Pensions, 2015)
- 68,110 children were looked after in England (Glendinning, 2013)
- 87,160 young people with proven offences and 1,834 young people were in custody in 2015 (Minstry of Justice, 2016)

Table I.2 Six perspectives of wellbeing

	Objective wellbeing	Objective and subjective wellbeing	Subjective wellbeing
Personal wellbeing	Focus on measurable observable wellbeing outcomes at the individual level.	Focus on a holistic range of wellbeing outcomes at the individual level.	Focus on experiences of subjective wellbeing at the individual level.
Personal and social wellbeing	Focus on measurable observable wellbeing outcomes at the individual level with social and environmental factors.	Focus on a holistic range of wellbeing outcomes at the individual level with social and environmental factors.	Focus on experiences of subjective wellbeing at the individual level with social and environmental factors.
Social wellbeing	Focus on measurable observable wellbeing outcomes at the social level.	Focus on a holistic range of wellbeing outcomes at the social level.	Focus on experiences of subjective wellbeing at the social level.

- 1 in 10 young people has mental health issues (Green et al., 2005)
- 60,940 families in temporary accommodation (Wilson, 2015)
- 3,510,555 young people are not in any form of education, training or employment (Office for National Statistics, 2014), reducing to 826,000 after the age of leaving school was increased by two years (Office for National Statistics, 2017).

What is perhaps lacking is evidence of the impact that these objective measures have on personal wellbeing. Whilst the relationship between poverty and subjective wellbeing has been explored, there is little to enable us to understand how being in care, living in temporary accommodation, living in custody or worklessness impact on subjective wellbeing. Still less understood is the extent to which poor subjective wellbeing can lead to crime, worklessness and so on. In this book we attempt to create a model that encompasses this complexity by locating personal wellbeing within social and environmental settings, and by valuing the objective and subjective equally.

The collection of statistics above also illuminates that wellbeing is not a single service issue. It is not the task of teachers, or social workers, or youth workers alone to tackle this complex issue. Rather it is a multi-agency response that is demanded. A multi-agency approach is primarily necessary due to the multi-faceted nature of wellbeing. A secondary driver in the UK has been the year on year cuts to statutory services, particularly at a time of increased need (especially relating to mental health) which has fostered new and unique partnerships. In particular, there have been increased demands of the voluntary and charitable sector and new partnerships between them and the statutory sector. Some of these changes have led to new role descriptions. Youth workers, for example, often find themselves in roles as 'key workers' or 'learning mentors', in an increasing hybridisation of professional roles.

Given the complexity already introduced of perspectives, definitions and multi-agency work, it is unsurprising that practitioners, managers and commissioners may find themselves confused as to what to do to best support wellbeing. In many countries, including the UK, there is no explicit practice or pedagogy of wellbeing.

Further, the pedagogy of the voluntary and community sector is often implicit and frameworks for practice tacit in our informal or non-formal approach. There is a new need to make this explicit; to articulate it and showcase it as a valid, robust and evidenced approach to bring to these new contexts and partnerships.

Our work, culminating in this book, tries to meet this need and better understand how practitioners work with CYPF to support wellbeing in this context.

This was based on the critical assumption that as practitioners *we can't do wellbeing to people*. You can't give a pill for wellbeing. This is not the same as in the mental health field, where medication is critiqued. Similarly, we can't make people well or fix them: tell them to feel good and function well. In our experience, as soon as we start to 'tell', the people, particularly those experiencing some of the negative and deprived conditions described earlier, either push back, or do not know how to sustain change. For this change is our (the practitioner's) perception of well, not the person's. Therefore, our argument is that CYPF wellbeing needs to be discovered and defined by them. It is an intrinsic process; it is experiential.

This perspective focuses the discussion onto how we support CYPF to discover how they feel good and function well. So then how do we work in this context? This distinguishes the power in the relationship to sit with the CYPF. It is not ours to give, it is theirs to grow and develop. This is a concept, whilst not new to some working with CYPF, is hugely challenging for others. It is supportive and facilitative; it can take time and resources; and it has been criticised for being woolly and un-robust. However, we happen to think that it is very robust, an art and a science. This book is our attempt at capturing this work into a robust framework for people to use to underpin their practice. It comes from multiple research projects focusing on practice and practitioners. It encompasses these into one common model that can be used as a common framework for those working with CYPF to support them to develop their wellbeing.

The key defining facet of this approach to developing wellbeing is looking at it through a social justice lens. This gives a new shape to the wellbeing discussion and a new lens to look at it through.

Social justice and wellbeing

As stated above, there is a link between disadvantage and a lack of wellbeing. This can also been seen as access to wellbeing. When considering wellbeing from this perspective we are speaking the language of social justice. Social justice refers to equity and equality within society. We emphasise here that there is a critical relationship between wellbeing and social justice. This asserts that there should be equity in access to feeling good and functioning well. However, there clearly is not this equity. People have equal rights to wellbeing, but because of their context and relative disadvantage, they do not. Conversely, those with access to assets and opportunity are more likely to achieve and have higher wellbeing. This is not a blanket statement, as of course there are cases that 'break the mould'.

This view is supported by social capital theory that maps the ways in which networks of relationships support CYPF to achieve positive outcomes (Putnam, 2000). Further, the more functional wellbeing (relating to agency) that CYPF have, the more likely they are to fight for their rights and those of others, creating a more socially just world, whereas those struggling to feed themselves may have limited opportunities to achieve personal, local, national or global change.

This leads to the assertion that our role as professionals is to support people's access to wellbeing, to support them to understand their rights and access resources to develop their own wellbeing. Here we can draw from critical pedagogy to help underpin our approach to supporting wellbeing.

Critical pedagogy and wellbeing

Critical pedagogy is a liberatory and developmental process that involves increased awareness, challenge, dialogue and social action. It is a pedagogy that provides an approach of supporting CYPF to develop their own wellbeing.

Critical pedagogy, and in particular the works of Paulo Freire (1973), argues that people need to become aware of their own oppression before they can change, learn, grow and develop. Freire outlined how people can be naïve with 'intransitive thought', rather than critically conscious. In this state, people lack insight into the way in which their social conditions undermine their wellbeing and so do not see their own actions as capable of changing their conditions (Campbell and MacPhail, 2002). Critical pedagogy is therefore an approach to social justice and thus wellbeing.

Structure and agency and wellbeing

When considering the different conditions CYPF are in, we draw in debates of structuralism. CYPF do not exist in a society free from control; they are surrounded by structures such as laws, rules, social norms, etc. These can both constrain and enable their agency. Agency is CYPF's ability to act. For example, the extent of freedom of speech in any society will influence the awareness of its people. The extent of judicial rules and social norms will affect the extent to which someone feels they can make choices, and the actions that they deem possible. This is not to say that people are entirely controlled by society – that is called a structuralist view (Durkheim, 1982).

We take time in this book therefore to identify structures, and to define agency. We position them as a dualism acting on one another, rather than as an opposing duality. This draws from both Giddens's (1994) structuration theory and Archer's (1995) double morphogenesis. When viewed in this way, structures enable and constrain the agency of CYPF and their actions act on and change or reinforce the structures. An individual or group will have varying degrees of ability to act on, or in, this structure. This is dynamic; ever changing and situational.

Coote (2010), in discussing the Big Society agenda of the, then, coalition government, describes that when people are given the chance and treated as if they are capable, they tend to find that they know what is best for themselves and can fix their own problems. She identifies this as underpinning any efforts to get more people working together to run their own affairs locally. This perspective is extended (albeit in a critique of the Big Society agenda) by Ledwith (2011) who states that when people *have control over what is happening in their lives (agency), their health and wellbeing improves*. This forms the fundamental assumption on which this book is based.

In defining agency as the ability that CYPF have to make choices and to act on them, amid differing contexts and structures (Stuart, 2013), our investigation deepens into our approach or pedagogy, for which we do this. A critical approach, or pedagogy, supports CYPF to be aware of themselves and their context, before they can act in/on it. This is through a process of empowerment.

Empowerment and wellbeing

Empowerment is a complex concept that is often reduced to oversimplified terms. Empowerment is about a person's sense of power. This includes personal and psychological power, discursive and cultural power. It incorporates the sense of power to, power over, power from, and power with and within. It includes multiple sources of power such as knowledge, roles, positions and assets. It is therefore another complex and multi-dimensional term (Thompson, 2007).

Again, empowerment cannot be done to CYPF. It is an intrinsic process and only something that can be done for themselves (Maynard, 2011). As professionals we can facilitate this process, providing conditions that may spark a process enabling CYPF to empower themselves. This is our central thesis within this book; our core model to help frame our practice of developing wellbeing. We define this process of empowerment in three clear phases:

- *Awareness* – this is a catalytic process, sparking new thought or realisation, the outcomes of which are increased consciousness of 'this is who I am', 'this is what I like and dislike' and 'this is what I am good at and not good at'.
- *Choice* – this is the drive from the spark leading to CYPF commitment to a change process, to commit to using personal power to achieve personal gain. This may be a positive move towards something as in 'I want that', or an avoidance of a negative outcome as in 'I don't want that!' Further, it leads to a belief in one's self, saying 'I can do that'.
- *Action* – this is actually taking the action and making change. This is informed, ongoing and sustained change. This is regarding oneself; both in and for society, as well as collective, for example when communities take action.

Our role here as professionals is to facilitate this process. This is an experiential process facilitating people's exploration by creating catalytic conditions to challenge the status quo and induce new ways of thinking, believing and behaving. Our central proposition is therefore that critical pedagogy is the process of facilitating empowerment and agency towards enhanced social justice and wellbeing.

Although this is not new to many practitioners, it is to some. However, what is new is the different ways we have to work – the different needs and issues, policies, funding conditions and partnerships. It is our practice(s) within these contemporary contexts that require a clear and joined up framework in which we can design, deliver, evaluate and articulate our programmes collectively, showing how we achieve change for and with CYPF.

Why this book?

This book aims to offer a theoretical and practical guide to organisations, projects and practitioners trying to facilitate social justice and wellbeing. We noticed a disconnect between abstract concepts of wellbeing and tangible practice with CYPF. This book bridges the theory-practice divide, offering a clear and definitive guide to concepts and practical activities to embed in practice. It is making the implicit explicit.

We independently became interested in understanding the concept of wellbeing. Lucy started her journey within her Doctoral studies which explored sexually exploited young women's empowerment. Kaz's interest came from her Doctoral studies into structure and agency – which either supports or detracts from wellbeing. We worked together at Brathay Trust, a youth development organisation, where we had increased opportunity to explore the practical methods which practitioners were employing to support CYPF wellbeing. Here we refined and developed our independent works from within practice. This was a process of many cycles of action research. This book is an opportunity to capture our findings from within practice and offer this back to practice, amid uncertainty and need for clarity of firm foundations for organisations and practitioners.

Lucy continues to develop this work within practice as Head of Research at Brathay Trust. Kaz now works at the University of Cumbria, responsible for degrees that prepare students to practice with children, young people and families. In this book we hope to present you with the theory and practice that you need to understand and apply empowerment and agency in a range of settings in developing wellbeing and social justice.

The contents of the book

The book has been written for a practice-based audience. This is not divisive against academia, more about accessibility and practicality. Our experience suggests that practitioners aren't concerned with peer reviewed referencing and some of the laws that govern our academic literature. They are interested in clear, concise and robust information that is rich in practice-based reality. Therefore, this is the pitch of this book: we want to switch practitioners on, not switch them off!

The book is designed so that you can read it cover to cover or dip in and out. To help those that prefer to 'dip', we have provided a guide to the contents of the different chapters. To this end there are also key point summaries at the end of each chapter.

We have broken this book down into sections: *what* the framework is, *where* we have seen it in practice and *how* you could employ it within your own practice. The first section of the book (the *what* section) discusses the thinking and theory behind the framework. It builds the framework, so it can be understood at multiple levels. The second section (the *where and how* section) provides case study examples of the framework. This is from a variety of practices which have either adopted the framework or we have observed and mapped on to the framework. The *how* section draws out specific skills and tools to engage with this approach to supporting CYPF wellbeing.

The two sections are linked, so as not to encourage a theory practice divide and exemplify praxis. There are vignettes in the theory sections to contextualise it and reference to theory in the case studies. These vignettes are of relevant policy, practice and research. There are also stimulus questions and tasks that will enable you to apply what you have just read to your practice. There is also a practice toolkit offered on Routledge's companion website to further enable you to embed these ideas into your daily work. Further reading is also signposted throughout the book to ensure that you can follow up on any of the ideas introduced.

Part 1

Chapter 1. Wellbeing and social justice

Wellbeing is introduced and the differences between wellbeing and other concepts, such as resilience, are discussed. Objective and subjective wellbeing will be described and different professional perspectives on wellbeing integrated. Wellbeing is introduced as operating in relationship with social justice and as interdependent. Therefore, increasing wellbeing also contributes to social justice and vice versa. Recent UK data is used to quantify the scale of the issues discussed, recent research is profiled, and vignettes bring the concepts to life in real terms.

Chapter 2. Wellbeing from multi-disciplinary perspectives

This chapter will critically compare and contrast the ways in which different professions view wellbeing. It illuminates similarities and differences based on each profession's construct of the 'child', 'young person', or 'family'. This draws from the multiple contexts we now find ourselves working within, including health, education, social care, policing and youth work.

Chapter 3. Wellbeing from global perspectives

Wellbeing is an international phenomenon. This chapter will explore the different ways in which wellbeing is conceptualised in policy terms and measured in different countries and compare measures of wellbeing internationally.

Chapter 4. Wellbeing and critical pedagogy

Critical pedagogy is a form of learning that promotes empowerment and agency, and so social justice. The roots and history of critical pedagogy are described and key theorists highlighted. Vignettes present critical pedagogy in practice and profile research that supports its use. The advantages and limitations of the approach are described. The majority of this chapter is devoted to describing critical pedagogical approaches that can be observed, planned and measured, making clear links between theory and practice.

Chapter 5. Wellbeing, structures and post-structuralism

Structuralism is described as the view that people are created by the environments and societies that they live in; they are structured by them. Examples of this form of thinking are profiled in vignettes and the theorists who lead this line of sociology are profiled. The benefits and limitations of the structuralist approach are identified.

Chapter 6. Wellbeing and agency

Agency is defined as CYPF ability to be aware of the world around them, to choose a course of action and to act on it, creating the world that they want. In this sense, agency is the state that people need to possess in order to have wellbeing and in order to create a more socially just world. Theorists who privilege this perspective present the view that people create societies (Giddens, Archer, Bandura). Both psychological and sociological perspectives are included. Examples of this form of thinking are profiled in vignettes and the theorists who lead this line of sociology are profiled. The benefits and limitations of the agentic approach are identified. The chapter concludes by presenting a balanced view of structure and agency as a dualism rather than as a duality.

Chapter 7. Wellbeing, empowerment and oppression

Empowerment is framed as a process where individuals and groups counter oppression. Empowerment is presented as the process by which people develop agency, it is the route to agency, and therefore wellbeing and social justice. Empowerment is not something that can be 'gifted' or 'bestowed' to people. We cannot 'do it' to other people, yet this is often how the word 'empowerment' is used in policy and practice. A framework for empowerment is described and illuminated by practice examples. The chapter concludes with a conceptual framework representing the relationship between wellbeing, social justice, empowerment and agency.

Part 2

The second section of the book provides case studies of empowerment and agency in practice and demonstrates practical ways to embed the ideas from the first half of the book into your practice. The settings of the case studies include:

Chapter 8. A critical pedagogical approach to tackling sexual exploitation

This case study is based on a three-year programme supporting young women who were being sexually exploited. The chapter describes how and why the young women were in this situation, highlighting the importance of awareness of structures. It traces the critical approach used within a mixed community and residential project and describes the impact for the group and individuals.

Chapter 9. A critical pedagogical approach to reducing re-offending

This chapter is based on a programme designed to reduce re-offending in a rural local authority. The case study examines the story of one young man on the programme who was living a high risk life, alcoholic, violent, workless, and in trouble with the police. The year-long programme provided structured personal development activities, sparked his realisation that his life could be different, and supported his empowerment with mentoring. Key points are made that a critical pedagogical approach can be a powerful tool for individual development, and that development is not linear, but cyclical.

Chapter 10. A critical pedagogical approach to learning and employability

This chapter describes a school-based programme supporting the wellbeing and resilience of young people. It aims to increase their engagement with learning and reduce their risk of offending and anti-social behaviour. The case study illuminates how awareness is the foundation of other personal and social outcomes that precede learning or pro-social behaviour.

Chapter 11. A critical pedagogical approach to homelessness

The Foyer Federation has 300 Foyers nationally that provide housing solutions and personal development for around 8000 young people a year in the UK. The support is planned and delivered from an asset-based perspective. This case study explores how the Foyer Federation used their organisational agency to launch this asset-based youth offer, and how the offer supports homeless young people from a critical pedagogical approach.

Chapter 12. A critical pedagogical approach to social action and leadership

This chapter explores a programme that supports young leaders of social enterprise – The Aspiring Leaders Programme or ALP. The programme is an interesting partnership between a youth work organisation (Brathay Trust) and University (The University of Cumbria) and is accredited with an undergraduate degree. The key assumption behind the programme is that aspiring leaders need support to be able to lead social action within their organisations and communities. Research on the project demonstrated that the aspiring leaders particularly needed support to develop resilience and this case study explores how that was achieved in a critically pedagogical way.

Chapter 13. A critical pedagogical approach to family work

This case study describes an approach to family learning that is rooted in critical pedagogy. The practitioner supporting this work has developed 'authentic family learning', bringing Freirian principles of authentic learning to a family learning setting. The case study explores how this work has been created and how families respond to this different way of working.

Chapter 14. A critical pedagogical approach to practitioner development

This case study explores the critical pedagogical approach used in action research exploring the leadership activity of leaders and managers in the children's workforce in one local authority (education, health, policing, social care, further education, family services). The case study shows that leaders and managers with high levels of critical consciousness have more agency as leaders, and secondly points to the role of reflection within an action research project in levering critical consciousness.

Chapter 15. Critical pedagogical practices

This chapter introduces a range of common critically pedagogical practices including: third spaces, dialogue, narratives, media critique, creative arts, authentic learning and philosophy for children. These are not comprehensive guides to each practice, rather they provide a conceptual overview, and idea of what they mean practically. The chapter signposts you to further resources and toolkits for each practice to ensure that you have somewhere else to deepen your understanding.

Conclusion

The conclusion refers back to the conceptual framework established and reiterates the link between wellbeing, social justice, empowerment and agency and the role of critically pedagogical practice. The conclusion draws the range of case studies together and links them to the conceptual framework. Practitioners are reminded that the practicalities of delivering work in a critical pedagogical manner demand a critical pedagogical approach. Empowerment and agency are argued to be concepts and practices that are multi-disciplinary, intergenerational, and equally applicable to practitioners as to 'service users'. They are both concepts that are argued to be vital to the wellbeing and social justice of people, communities, the UK and global population and therefore worth their efforts to deliver.

For us, wellbeing and social justice are the fundamental contemporary issues. We believe that life should be a positive experience for everyone. The apparent complexity of wellbeing, the range of rhetoric and lack of practical guides on the subject, have motivated us to write this text.

Because wellbeing is a subject addressed by a wide range of professions, we believe that the book is relevant to:

- Teaching
- Informal education
- Outdoor education
- Social work
- Youth work
- Youth offending work
- Health care
- Family support
- Community development.

The combination of theory and practice ideas we hope makes the book appropriate to all stages of career development. It supports students and practitioners who work with CYPF to embed critical pedagogy in their practice supporting wellbeing. It also provides a practice-driven frame of reference to critically engage in policy analysis. It offers leaders and managers a new perspective on their organisations and interventions, and raises questions for further research for academics.

We hope that you enjoy reading it.

Key terms

We use the following four words as verbal short cuts throughout the book:

CYPF: an acronym for children, young people and families. Children and young people live within peer groups, families and communities, therefore important to consider working with them in each of these settings.

Professional/practitioner: all practitioners are professionals in our minds. We do not limit our thinking to judgements about professional status. The terms professional and practitioner are therefore used interchangeably and without prejudice.

Practice: we refer to practice in the singular, but please keep your mind open and think of individual, group, family and community based practice.

Wellbeing: as we have started to assert above, and continue in the next chapter, wellbeing and social justice are interrelated concepts. However, we often refer to just wellbeing as a shorter phrase. Where we refer only to wellbeing, we are coming from a perspective that includes social justice, as our position is that the two are inextricably related.

References

Aked, J., Marks, N., Cordon, C., and Thompson, S. (2008). *Five Ways to Wellbeing: The Evidence*. London: nef.

Archer, M. (1995). *Realist Social Theory: The Morphogenetic Approach*. Cambridge: Cambridge University Press.

Bandura, A. (2001). 'Social Cognitive Theory: An Agentic Perspective', *Annual Review of Psychology*, 51, 1–26.

Campbell, C., and MacPhail, C. (2002). 'Peer Education, Gender and the Development of Critical Consciousness: Participatory HIV Prevention by South African Youth', *Social Science and Medicine*, 55(2), 331–345.

Coote, A. (2010). *Ten Big Questions About the Big Society and Ten Ways to Make the Best of It*. London: nef.

Department for Education and Skills (DfES) (2004). *Every Child Matters: Change for Children*. London: DfES.

Department for Education and Skills (DfES) (2005). *Youth Matters*. Cm 6629. London: HMSO.

Department for Work and Pensions (DWP) (2015) *Low Income Statistics: Lowest Levels Since 1980s*. Accessed on 22. 4. 17 at: https://www.gov.uk/government/news/low-income-statistics-lowest-levels-since-1980s

Durkheim, E. (1982). *The Rules of Sociological Method*. New York: Free Press. European Society of Endocrinology. (2011). 'New method to measure cortisol could lead to better understanding of development of common diseases', *ScienceDaily*, May 3, 2011. Accessed on 2/9/16 at: www.sciencedaily.com/releases/2011/05/110502183715.htm

Freire, P. (1973). *Education for a Critical Consciousness*. New York: Seabury Press.

Giddens, A. (1994). *Beyond the Left and the Right, the Future of Radical Politics*. Cambridge: Polity Press.

Glendinning, C. (2013) 'Long Term Care Reform in England: A Long and Unfinished Story', in Ranci, C. and Pavolini, E. (eds) *Reforms in Long Term Care Policies in Europe: Investigating Institutional Change and Social Impacts*. New York: Springer, pp. 179–200.

Green, H., McGinnity, A., Meltzer, H., Ford, T., and Goodman, R. (2005). *Mental Health of Children and Young People in Great Britain: 2004*. London: Office for National Statistics.

Henderson, S., Holland, J., McGrellis, S., Sharpe, S., and Thomson, R. (2007). *Inventing Adulthoods. A Biographical Approach to Youth Transitions*. London: Sage Publications.

Layard, R. (2002) *Happiness: Has Social Science Got a Clue?* Accessed 1/4/15 at: http://cep.lse.ac.uk/events/lectures/layard/RL030303.pdf

Ledwith, M. (2011). *Community Development a Critical Approach*. London: Policy Press.

Margo, J., and Sodha, S. (2007). *Get Happy: Children and Young People's Emotional Wellbeing*. London: NCH.

Maynard, L. (2011). '"Suddenly I See" Outdoor Youth Development's Impact on Young Women's Well-Being: A Model of Empowerment'. PhD Thesis. Lancaster University.

Michaelson, J., Abdallah, S., Steuer, N., Thompson, S., and Marks, N. (2009). *National Accounts of Well-being: Bringing Real Wealth onto the Balance Sheet*. London: nef.

Ministry of Justice (2016). *Youth Justice Statistics 2014–15*. London: Ministry of Justice and Youth Justice Board.

Office for National Statistics (2014). *Statistical Bulletin: Young People Not in Education, Employment or Training (NEET) 2014*. Accessed on 22. 4. 17 at: https://www.ons.gov.uk/employmentandlabourmarket/peoplenotinwork/unemployment/bulletins/youngpeoplenotineducationemploymentortrainingneet/2015-08-20

Office for National Statistics (2017). *Statistical Bulletin: Young People Not in Education, Employment or Training (NEET) 2017*. Accessed on 22. 4. 17 at: https://www.ons.gov.uk/employmentandlabourmarket/peoplenotinwork/unemployment/bulletins/youngpeoplenotineducationemploymentortrainingneet/feb2017#total-young-people-who-were-neet

Public Health England (2015). *Improving Young People's Health and Wellbeing: A Framework for Public Health*. London: PHE.

Putnam, R. (2000). *Bowling Alone: The Collapse and Revival of American Community*. New York: Simon and Schuster.

Stuart, K. (2013). 'Collaborative Agency Across Professional and Organisational Boundaries in the Children's Workforce in the UK'. PhD Thesis. Lancaster University.

The Children's Society (2013). *The Good Childhood Report*. London: The Children's Society.

Thompson, N. (2007). *Power and Empowerment*. Lyme Regis: Russell House Publishing.

White, S., Gaine, S., Jha, S. (2012). 'Beyond Subjective Well-being: A Critical Review of the Stiglitz Report Approach to Subjective Perspectives on Quality of Life', *International Development*, 24(6), 763–776.

Wilson, W. (2015). *Homeless Households in Temporary Accommodation*. London: House of Commons Library.

Part 1

Empowerment and agency: a critical theoretical framework to support practice

1   Wellbeing and social justice

Chapter overview

Wellbeing was defined in the introduction as comprising both objective and subjective factors, viewed differently by a range of professionals. In this chapter we propose that a focus on social justice is the key way to support wellbeing – and that without social justice, there will be no lasting wellbeing – the two are interdependent. An overview and discussion of different conceptualisations of social justice is presented with their resonance with wellbeing.

Unusually we are going to start this chapter with an activity.

Reflective activity: key task

What do you understand social justice to be?

How would you describe it to a board of trustees/directors/senior managers?

How would you describe it to the people that you work with – colleagues and CYPF?

Now read the description of different types of social justice below and see how your understanding fits.

The theoretical and practical work of social justice can be seen as a response to injustice. Injustice takes a wide range of forms, and consequently, people who talk about or practice social justice can have very different foci. However, social justice is concerned with the just distribution of wealth, the right to justice through social control, the just access of opportunity, a moral obligation, and what we call functional social justice. As you might expect, amid this range, there are many definitions. For example, Chapman and West-Burnham (2010) outline,

Equality: every human being has an absolute and equal right to common dignity and parity of esteem and entitlement to access the benefits of society on equal terms.

Equity: every human being has a right to benefit from the outcomes of society on the basis of fairness and according to need.

Therefore, *social justice* requires deliberate and specific intervention to secure equality and equity.

Some people think that achieving social justice is a utopian dream. Neo-liberal advocates will say that social justice is impossible and would destroy market forces and the global economy. It is interesting to note, therefore, that countries with a deep commitment to social justice also have the highest level of wellbeing – namely Japan, Sweden, Finland, Norway, Denmark and the Netherlands (Chapman and West-Burnham, 2010: 28). This is exemplified further in the vignette below.

Vignette 1.1 Social Justice in Sweden

The Social Justice in Europe Index Report (Schraad-Tischler, 2015) measured indicators on poverty prevention, equitable education, labour market access, social cohesion and non-discrimination, health and intergenerational justice in its weightings.

Some top and bottom five results are shown below. The scores are all out of 10:

1st	Sweden	7.23
2nd	Denmark	7.10
3rd	Finland	7.02
4th	Netherlands	6.84
5th	Czech Republic	6.68
23rd	Hungary and Spain	4.73
25th	Italy	4.69
26th	Bulgaria	3.78
27th	Romania	3.74
28th	Greece	3.61
European Average:		5.63

(Adapted from the Bertelsmann Foundation, 2015: 1).

Sweden, the most socially just country in the rankings, holds its position for some of the following reasons:

- It has the most diverse national parliament (45% female)
- Only 9.8% of young people in Sweden were NEET compared to a 17.8% EU average (ibid, 139–141).
- Only 1.1% of Swedes work long hours compared to 12.5% of workers in European countries

- 88.2% of the adult working age population of Sweden have completed at least an upper secondary education compared to the European average of 77.2%
- Sweden's voter turnout stands at 85.8% compared to the European average of 68.4%
- Only 1.6% of children in Sweden are obese, lower than the European average of 2.7% (OECD, 2015).

Whilst social justice may be cited as a utopian dream that is not possible in a neo-liberal world, Sweden seems to be managing pretty well.

Whilst you may be able to compare one country to another, or one school to another and say one is more socially just than another, social justice itself is something that is either present or absent. Any given context will either feature injustice or social justice.

Nevertheless, social justice is also a highly dynamic state and is situational. It may exist in some contexts and not in others. It may exist in some countries, communities, organisations or classrooms, but not in others. How people act, minute by minute, will influence and affect social justice. The way we address young people may vary from day to day and will be an example of the equity and equality available at that moment.

However, this is not only a global, social or political agenda. It is a personal and interpersonal agenda. In our own small way we all create a greater social justice in the world around us, like casting pebbles in a pond. This is particularly important to those of us who work to support CYPF wellbeing. If we don't consider this work within context, more specifically considering their equity and equality, then our work is at risk of being disassociated, abstract, unsustainable or redundant. This illuminates the perspective that the personal is both social and political and our work therefore needs to be considered as such.

Further, social justice is not contained as a theory or principle alone, social justice is a way of working and engaging with CYPF. This perspective urges you to combine theory and practice into praxis – the use of theory and practice together. We advocate for you to understand the theories of social justice and bring them to life vividly in your daily activities working with CYPF.

Dimensions of social justice

Having established the importance of social justice, and what is meant by the term overall, we will now explore the five dimensions of social justice.

Social Justice as the equal distribution of resources

Social justice, in one sense, refers to the just distribution of wealth and resources in society. Poverty remains a global issue, and a shocking issue even within the so-called developed western nations. For many, social justice is focused on making the distribution of wealth and resources more just.

To ensure a just distribution, many societies have engaged in the redistribution of wealth. Taxation is one example of State attempts to redistribute wealth. Taxing the rich funds social welfare benefits for those in need, along with central services such as education and health care for all. Social workers and family support workers may work within this perspective accessing welfare support for their clients and supporting them to get the benefits they are due from the State.

Whilst this redistribution may lead to a fairer society (Rawls, 1971), recent data is showing that the wealth gap is ever widening in the 21st century (Wilkinson and Pickett, 2010). It would seem therefore to only have a limited impact on justice. The redistribution approach also tends to ignore the conditions that led to the injustice occurring in the first place (Young, 1990).

From a global perspective the contrasts in resources and relative power bases held by organisations vary. Rich countries dominate poorer ones; those with bountiful resources call the shots when others run low and recent refugee crises push international perspectives of social justice and inclusion. These international situations really illustrate the relative power and powerlessness of the possession and control of resources on an individual level. These relative positions of power and powerlessness are replicated at a national and local level. In the UK, for example, there are projects that give free meals to young people throughout the summer holidays when they cannot access free school meals. The presence of food banks for families, free school meals and free holiday meal schemes emphasises the disparity between those that have and do not have money in the UK.

Social Justice and social control

This dimension of social justice focuses on "creating and maintaining social stability and order by exercising control over those who threaten to disrupt these" (Newman and Yeates, 2008: 13). The establishment of socially accepted norms of behaviour usually occurs through the process of socialisation. As children grow up they unconsciously notice and adhere to what is OK and not OK. This is sometimes reinforced explicitly through explanation, reward and punishment, and is also reinforced unconsciously through gossip, stories and media portrayal of 'heroes' and 'demons' within society. The judgements made within families, communities and societies become norms by which people self-regulate, and this creates a system of informal social control. This begs the question, what happens when people do not adhere to the rules?

The criminal justice system is in place to enforce social control when social norms are breached on a grand scale. The presence of the criminal justice system and its laws creates social control merely by its existence, and when those laws are breached then social control is enforced by punishment through financial fines or imprisonment. This type of social justice is for the masses. The criminal justice system is protecting the masses from the errant ways of individuals. Whilst judicial processes strive to be fair, there is a wealth of evidence on the criminalising effect of being in the criminal justice system (Whittaker, 2015) and of the over-representation of a range of oppressed and vulnerable groups (Roberts, 2016). This position suggests that the criminal justice system unintentionally can oppress and marginalise people. Policing, criminology and youth offending teams are likely to be working to this model of social justice.

Social Justice as freedom from discrimination

Nancy Fraser (1995) argues that social justice is more than access to resources, and highlights the importance of being seen as equally of worth in society. This depends on a variety of conditions, ranging from policy, access to education, to how people treat one another, and of particular relevance in today's society, how they are represented in the media and popular culture. This can encompass three areas:

- Forms and processes of discrimination
- The provision of equal opportunities and inclusion
- Social mobility.

Each is discussed in turn below.

Forms and processes of discrimination

Discrimination comes in many forms – sexism, racism, homophobia, classism, intellectualism, size-ism, to name a few. Fraser (1995) points out that it is usually those who are without resources who are also stereotyped and prejudiced against by society. People are multi-dimensional. Being a female is not Kaz's only feature, she is, for example also White British, an atheist, an academic, heterosexual, tattooed, etc. Discrimination and marginalisation can therefore relate to a range of things about us, at which point it becomes even more potent.

The discrimination can be seen as primary injury or hurt experienced by an individual. This is then reinforced by the lived experience of oppression and injustice, feelings of humiliation or anger or despair, what Bourdieu (1999) called 'social suffering'. People in society will react to the individual, perhaps avoiding young people in hoodies labelled as 'anti-social', looking down on the sexually exploited young woman labelled as 'asking for it', or shouting at refugees viewed as 'benefit thieves'. These labels and practices keep people in society safe as normal human beings, distant from these 'others'. Whilst abnormal people can be defined as 'other' there is no risk of becoming one of them. 'Othering' (Hoggett, 2001) and 'social abjection' (Tyler, 2013) are processes by which we keep ourselves safe and position other people in society as dangerous. Similarly, adopting a 'wilful blindness' (Heffernan, 2012) as we walk past the homeless, prevents us from recognising and relating to the issue, prevents us from seeing the injustice and having to act on it. These processes create a secondary harm, one perhaps more potent than the first experience of injustice. These acts say 'I don't see you', 'you don't matter', 'it's all your fault', and 'I don't care'.

Clarke (2008: 31) describes the processes of normalising and contesting different inequalities at different times and places as a deeply political and socio-cultural process. Whilst society is at liberty to ignore or condemn some people, other forms of discrimination have now become crimes, such as sexism. Which forms of discrimination are considered as illegal is interesting in its own right, as is the extent to which a law will curtail that form of societal behaviour. The use of the law to prohibit certain forms of discrimination further links this dimension of social justice to those of social control discussed earlier, and equal opportunity discussed next.

Equal opportunities and inclusion

Unless people are viewed equally, there will be no equality of access. It is only in relatively recent history that women have gained the vote worldwide, homosexuality is still illegal in some countries, some American states remain deeply racist, and disability rights vary worldwide. In other words, gender, sexuality, race and disability remain sources of discrimination in the world. People whose rights are not legitimised by the state typically stand a lesser chance of health, education, employment, participating in political processes and thriving for their own wellbeing (Beatty *et al.*, 2015: 32–34).

Social equality and equality of rights has been transformed into the political speak of social exclusion. As presented by New Labour in the UK, "the idea of social exclusion directs attention to the personal characteristics of the excluded rather than to the structures generating exclusion" (Lund, 2002: 206). This is further alluded to within the vignette below. This can easily lead to the creation of a moral underclass rather than a more inclusive society. The potential for stigmatisation increased with the range of groups identified at risk of social exclusion by the 2001 Social Exclusion Unit: rough sleepers, young runaways, prisoners, teenage mothers, low income families, drug addicts and deprived neighbourhoods.

Social mobility

Social mobility refers to the ability (and therefore, enablers and disablers) of people to move between layers of a stratified society, upwards or downwards. The presence of social mobility is a pathway to greater equality as it means that unjust positions in society are not fixed but open to change. Social mobility may be experienced by an individual who has a significant career trajectory, or inter-generationally as a family becomes more highly educated generation after generation.

Social mobility has been considered low in the UK. As a result of this the UK Government has created a social mobility index (Social Mobility and Child Poverty Commission, 2016). This "compares the chances that a child from a disadvantaged background will do well at school and get a good job across each of the 324 local authority district areas of the UK" (2016: 5). The 2016 study found that young people in London experienced more social mobility than the rest of the country. Further, coastal areas, industrial areas, cities and affluent areas offered the least mobility. David Cameron's 'one nation' speech (Cameron, 2015) promised stronger families, a first class education system and well-paid jobs in order to increase social mobility. Somewhat ironically, family support was offered through the stigmatising 'Troubled Families Programme', educational support through the creation of privatised academies, and well-paid jobs by increases to the personal tax threshold. These could all be equally positioned as oppressive or marginalising practices rather than those that lever social mobility. This is exemplified further within the vignette below.

Thankfully, charitable organisations also support social mobility. Many do so indirectly through work targeted at a range of disadvantages, and others more explicitly. The Social Mobility Foundation (2016), for example, provides practical support for young people from low-income backgrounds to gain qualifications and work that might normally be outside their reach.

The presence or absence of social mobility may be considered an additional form of discrimination, linking with the start of this discussion. It also overlaps with other dimensions of social justice, as it is itself a form of social control, and governs the redistribution of wealth.

Vignette 1.2 The UK Social Justice Policy

In 2012 the UK Government published its first explicit policy on social justice called Social Justice Transforming Lives. The opening paragraphs of the policy set out the Government's view of social justice:

Social Justice is about making society function better – providing the support and tools to help turn lives around. This is a challenging new approach to tackling poverty in all its forms. It is not a narrative about income poverty alone: this Government believes that the focus on income over the last decades has ignored the root causes of poverty, and in doing so has allowed social problems to deepen and become entrenched (HM Government, 2012: 5).

The policy describes the following set of principles informing the approach:

1 A focus on prevention and early intervention
2 Where problems arise, concentrating interventions on recovery and independence, not maintenance

3   Promoting work for those who can as the most sustainable route out of poverty, while offering unconditional support to those who are severely disabled and cannot work
4   Recognising that the most effective solutions will often be designed and delivered at a local level
5   Ensuring that interventions provide a fair deal for the taxpayer

The policy relates social justice to another Government priority of increasing social mobility. It describes this related strategy to be about ensuring people are able to move up the social ladder, regardless of background. They relate this social justice strategy to ensuring everybody can put a foot on that ladder.

This policy has been criticised for the colonisation and misuse of common conceptual terms to advantage political positions. The opening sentence of this policy claims that "Social Justice is about making society function better – providing the support and tools to help turn lives around". This is not a definition of social justice. There is no mention of equality, equity or freedom from discrimination. The term is misappropriated to refer to a society that 'functions well'; leaving the reader to question if this means a society that adheres to the status quo. Social justice is not about "providing the support and tools to help turn lives around", it is about changing the living conditions, the social rules, societal norms and common practices so that everyone experiences a fair and just life. By supporting people, governments can potentially perpetuate disadvantage and reinforce discrimination.

Examination of each of the five key actions to support social justice from the UK Government perspective is equally demoralising. Early prevention and intervention can only be effective if they intervene early in the conditions that contribute to unjust lives. Attempting to prevent the damage done by unjust societies is like stopping the leaking dam with a finger.

Promoting recovery and independence sounds reassuring unless it translates into people exiting services rapidly as resources are withdrawn. And rather than dealing with recovery, it would be better to create a society that promotes thriving rather than conditions that people need to recover from.

The third statement asserts that work is the "most sustainable route out of poverty". This leaves the reader wondering "sustainable for whom?" If more people work then the UK budget would be more sustainable as fewer benefits would be needed. But if there are no increases in jobs, then being in a job will not necessarily be sustainable for employees. Without significant support, how will people in poverty compete for jobs against the well-to-do? Without a stable economy, how will organisations provide and sustain well-paid jobs for all the unemployed in the UK?

The notion of "effective solutions will often be designed and delivered at a local level" is a notion carried forward from the Big Society (Cabinet Office, 2010). Whilst it sounds like an empowering and participatory approach, it may also be read as an attempt by the government to shed responsibility and reduce resources as people in communities step up to fulfil state duties.

The final point, providing a fairer deal for tax payers is a faintly veiled reference to the UK Government's intent to stop 'benefit scroungers' who were perceived to unfairly take tax payers' money. This point hailed the 'Universal Credit', a single benefit which was stated to bring simple and fair benefits to those that needed them, but in practice has been found to further disadvantage those who are most in need (Citizens Advice Bureau, 2012).

Social Justice as a moral obligation

Writing from a Catholic social teaching perspective, Novak and Adams (2015) introduce the moral dimension to social justice. If we view people in society as interdependent then we must subscribe to our moral obligation to support one another. They state "our flourishing as humans depends on our developing certain social virtues and recognising our dependence on and duty to others in our continued vulnerability" (2015: 7). This reframes social justice as a way of thinking rather than as a state of affairs. As a way of thinking, we would all extend a civic duty to those not as well off as ourselves. We would extend our help to refugees, support rather than step over the homeless and offer care rather than curses to young offenders. As Benestad (2011: 151) states: "A just society depends on virtuous citizens".

The departure from morals may also be a tension for practitioners in helping professions. Novak and Adams (2015) point out that the rise of bureaucratic responses to human crises reduces the scope of the Social Worker to respond in a flexible, wise, moral way (2015: 246). Instead, they have to follow the book, particularly with an oversized case load. The de-professionalisation of Teaching, Social Work and other sectors may increasingly erode the relationships between client and practitioner and remove the moral duty that led practitioners into those value laden roles.

A functional view of social justice

Social justice comprises the different dimensions discussed. These are inter-related and unable to be tackled in isolation (Barry, 2005: 14). When all five dimensions of social justice are present, it is likely that people will experience wellbeing and function well. The presupposition is that when resources are distributed equally, when there is appropriate social control, when there is freedom from discrimination, and when there is a moral duty to others, then people will be able to be *more* well and function *better*. Social justice is therefore not just about creating the conditions for equity and equality, but also about enabling people to have capacity and capability to use their resources, opportunities and freedoms (*UK Equalities Review*, DCLG, 2007: 126). This therefore leads us to a definition of social justice as:

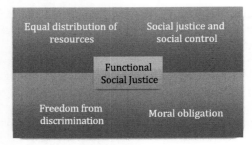

Figure 1.1 The dimensions of functional social justice

Social justice is a dynamic state of equality and equity present in any given situation, and people's ability to use their resources, opportunities and freedoms.

An injustice in one of these four areas can have profound impact on individuals and communities. A continued lack of social justice can also become self-sustaining as, for example, the experience of failing at school may teach a child that they are subordinate and unworthy, reducing their self-esteem and creating other social issues. This is exacerbated further by league tables and quantitative judgements of academic success, mechanisms that equate the 'less capable' with less important (Chapman and West-Burnham, 2010: 13–15). These injustices erode wellbeing. This leads to our central argument that social justice and wellbeing are inextricably linked. Our assumption is that if countries are socially just, then there is a high probability that CYPF will experience wellbeing (Chapman and West-Burnham, 2010: 30). This assertion has increasingly been supported by global data, as will be further explored in chapter 3.

Some have described the continued combination of these injustices as radical injustice (Pogge, 2004: 266–267). Radical injustice is defined by eight factors:

1   The worse off are very badly off in absolute terms
2   They are also very badly off in relative terms – they are very much worse off than many others
3   The inequality is impervious – it is difficult or impossible for the worse-off to substantially improve their lot. Most of the better off never experience life at the bottom for even a few months and have no vivid idea of what it is to live in that way
4   The inequality is pervasive – it concerns not merely some aspects of life, such as the climate, access to natural beauty, high culture; but all or most aspects
5   The inequality is avoidable – the better off can improve the circumstances of the worse off without becoming badly off themselves
6   There is a shared institutional order that is shaped by the better off and imposed on the worse off

7   This institutional order is implicated in the reproduction of radical inequality in that there is a feasible institutional alternative under which such severe and extensive inequality would not persist
8   The radical inequality cannot be traced to extra-social factors (such as genetic handicaps or natural disasters) which, as such, affect different human beings differently.

A single person cannot overthrow the system described by Pogge above, especially when the interests of the powerful are at risk within such an endeavour. Groups and communities can, however, enact social justice themselves within their communities, and can collectively bring about social change. This book is designed as a support for this critical practice – critically important and critically pedagogical.

Reflective activity

What different definitions of social justice exist in your workplace?
To what extent are you able to promote social justice in your workplace?
How socially just is your workplace?

Functional social justice and functional wellbeing

The functional view of social justice is in relationship with the functional view of wellbeing (remembering wellbeing is feeling good and functioning well). That is not to reject the other/single dimensions of social justice. Just as the functional view of wellbeing incorporated the subjective, objective, emotional, physical and psychological domains of wellbeing, so the functional view of social justice incorporates the dimensions of redistribution, inclusion, social control and moral duty.

Achieving social justice is therefore about supporting CYPF to function well. As social justice is a dynamic state, we can support increased equality and equity in terms of access to money, food, jobs, health, social status etc., leading to increased likelihood that CYPF will experience wellbeing.

This is important, because the more well CYPF are, the greater their ability to seek the equality and equity that they are due and the greater their ability to contribute to social justice themselves by ensuring resources are distributed equally, behaving fairly, acting without discrimination, and fulfilling their moral duty to others. Work needs to be done to both create socially just societies (the preconditions for wellbeing) and to support CYPF to be able to champion social justice. As Coote (2010) asserts, if people can support their own subjective and relative wellbeing then this will lead to improvements in absolute wellbeing through social change.

Rather than locating wellbeing as an issue that people need to solve individually, the functional approach keeps our minds open to the need to remove structural barriers to wellbeing present in society as well as supporting people to be in control of their own wellbeing (Widdowson, 2008: 67). We need to be ever mindful that we cannot give wellbeing to people, nor is it something that we can do for people; we can only support them to achieve this for themselves.

The danger of a personal responsibility approach is that the State may use this as a reason to withhold benefits if the claimant does not meet set conditions such as attending job interviews. This is problematic if it means people living below the poverty line have benefits stopped. The controversy over this issue triggered a Parliamentary review and on-going debate in the UK (House of Commons, 2015). This is in practice in the UK with unemployment benefits withheld from claimants if they do not adhere to a strict behavioural contract (Joseph Rowntree Foundation, 2014). This policy has been criticised as the employment contract is disempowering and so is an appropriation of the concept of functional wellbeing and personal autonomy matched with financial support.

Summary of key points

Social justice is more than a theory; it is a lived experience and a practice. Social justice comprises different dimensions, which need to be considered as functioning in interrelation so that we can support CYPF's increased wellbeing: feeling good and functioning well. Functional social justice contributes to wellbeing. When people are well, they are able to contribute to social justice.

The term social justice has recently been colonised for political purposes, and we need to read social justice policy with a critical eye to understand the extent to which it does what it claims to.

One could be forgiven for seeing a gloomy portrayal of social injustice in the world and asking what hope is there? However, as previously outlined, wellbeing has been found to improve when people have control over what is happening in their lives (Ledwith, 2011). Approaches that give control (power) back to individuals are therefore significant levers of wellbeing. This leads to the fundamental theoretical construct of this book that wellbeing is in relationship with social justice. They are contingent on one another as summarised in the diagram below.

This book presupposes that there is hope, and that hope lies in people like you working in a critically pedagogical way with communities and groups supporting their empowerment and agency and enabling them to experience greater wellbeing and to challenge the conditions that led to their unjust experiences in the first place. This is therefore a political process: our work is inherently political as we strive to influence and for the CYPF we work with to influence. These core principles are found in the chapters to follow.

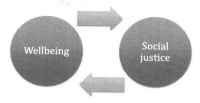

Figure 1.2 The relationship between wellbeing and social justice

Further reading

Chapman, L. and West-Burnham, J. (2010). *Education for Social Justice. Achieving Wellbeing for All*. London: Continuum.

Newton, J. and Yeates, N. (eds.) (2008) *Social Justice: Welfare, Crime and Society*. Maidenhead: Open University Press.

Tyler, I. (2013). *Revolting Subjects: Social Abjection and Resistance in Neoliberal Britain*. London: Zen Books.

Wilkinson, R. and Pickett, K. (2010). *The Spirit Level*. London: Sage

References

Barry, B. (2005). *Why Social Justice Matters*. Cambridge: Polity Press.

Beatty, C., Foden, M., McCarthy, L., and Reeve, K. (2015). *Benefit Sanctions and Homelessness: A Scoping Report*. Sheffield: Crisis and Sheffield Hallam University.

Benestad, B. (2011). *Church, State and Society*. New York: Catholic University of America Press.

Bourdieu, P. (1999). *The Weight of the World: Social Suffering in Contemporary Society*. Cambridge: Polity.

Cabinet Office (2010). *Building the Big Society*. London: Cabinet Office.

Cameron, D. (2015). 'One Nation Speech'. Accessed 22. 4. 16 at https://www.gov.uk/government/speeches/pm-speech-on-opportunity

Chapman, L., and West-Burnham, J. (2010). *Education for Social Justice. Achieving Wellbeing for All*. London: Continuum.

Citizens Advice Bureau (2012). 'Citizens Advice outlines its concerns on the Universal Credit'. Accessed 22. 4. 16 at https://www.citizensadvice.org.uk/about-us/how-citizens-advice-works/media/press-releases/citizens-advice-outlines-its-concerns-on-the-new-universal-credit/

Clarke, J. (2008). 'Looking for Social Justice, Welfare States and Beyond' in Newton, J., and Yeates, N. (eds.) *Social Justice: Welfare, Crime and Society*. Maidenhead: Open University Press, pp. 29–62.

Coote, A. (2010). *Ten Big Questions About the Big Society and Ten Ways to Make the Best of It*. London: nef.

Department of Communities and Local Government (DCLG) (2007) *UK Equalities Review*. London: DCLG.

Fraser, N. (1995). *Justice Interruptus. Critical Reflections on the 'Postsocialist' Condition*. London: Routledge.

Heffernan, M. (2012). *Wilful Blindness: Why We Ignore the Obvious*. London: Simon and Schuster.

HM Government (2012). *Social Justice: Transforming Lives.* London: HMSO.

Hoggett, P. (2001). 'Agency, Rationality and Social Policy', *Journal of Social Policy*, 30(1), 37–56.

House of Commons (2015). *Benefit Sanctions Policy: Beyond the Oakley Review.* Accessed on 22. 4. 17 at: https://www.publications.parliament.uk/pa/cm201415/cm select/cmworpen/814/814.pdf

Joseph Rowntree Foundation (2014). *Welfare Sanctions and Conditionality in the UK.* London: JRF. Accessed on 4/9/16 at: https://www.jrf.org.uk/sites/default/files/jrf/m igrated/files/Welfare-conditionality-UK-Summary.pdf

Ledwith, M. (2011). *Community Development a Critical Approach.* London: Policy Press.

Lund, B. (2002). *Understanding State Welfare: Social Justice or Social Exclusion?* London: Sage.

Newman, J., and Yeates, N. (2008). 'Introduction', in Newton, J. and Yeates, N. (eds) *Social Justice: Welfare, Crime and Society.* Maidenhead: Open University Press, pp. 1–24.

Novak, M., and Adams, P. (2015). *Social Justice Isn't What You Think It Is.* New York: Encounter Books.

OECD (2015). *How's Life in Sweden?* Paris: OECD.

Pogge, T. (2004). 'Brief for a Global Resources Dividend', in Clayton, M. and Williams, A. (eds) *Social Justice.* Oxford: Blackwell Publishing.

Rawls, J. (1971). *A Theory of Justice.* Cambridge, MA: Harvard University Press.

Roberts, R. (2016). *Racism and Criminal Justice.* Centre for Criminal Justice Studies. Accessed on 4/9/16 at: https://www.crimeandjustice.org.uk/publications/cjm/article/ racism-and-criminal-justice

Schraad-Tischler, D. (2015). *Social Justice in the EU – Index Report 2015. Social Inclusion Monitor Europe.* Accessed on 22. 4. 17 at: https://www.bertelsmann-stiftung.de/fileadm in/files/BSt/Publikationen/GrauePublikationen/Studie_NW_Social-Justice-in-the-EU- Index-Report-2015_2015.pdf

Social Mobility and Child Poverty Commission (2016) *Social Mobility Index.* London: HMSO.

Social Mobility Foundation (2016). *Overview.* Accessed on 23. 4. 16 at http://www. socialmobility.org.uk/about-us/#content

Tyler, I. (2013). *Revolting Subjects: Social Abjection and Resistance in Neoliberal Britain.* London: Zen Books.

Widdowson, B. (2008). 'Well-being, Harm and Work', in Newton, J. and Yeates, N. (eds) *Social Justice: Welfare, Crime and Society.* Maidenhead: Open University Press, pp. 134–156.

Wilkinson, R., and Pickett, K. (2010). *The Spirit Level.* London: Sage.

Whittaker, L. (2015). *Criminal Justice in the United Kingdom 2010–2015: Criminalising Poverty.* Open University Open Learn. Accessed on 4/9/16 at: http://www.open.edu/ openlearn/people-politics-law/the-law/criminology/criminal-justice-the-united-kingdom- 2010-2015-criminalising-poverty

Young, L. (1990). *Justice and the Politics of Difference.* Princeton, NJ: Princeton University Press.

2 Wellbeing from multi-disciplinary perspectives

Chapter overview

This chapter will compare and contrast the ways in which different professions view wellbeing including health, education, social care, policing and youth work. These differences arise from each profession's construct of the child, the young person, the family, or indeed the community. The chapter goes on to consider how organisational development considers wellbeing, and how the wellbeing of professionals is as important as that of CYPF they are trying to support.

Multi-disciplinary perspectives

A discipline is a particular type of work with a strong history and philosophy of training. Medicine, or healthcare, is an example of a discipline. A discipline is very broad and often has a range of different professional roles within it. For example, in healthcare there are GPs, radiologists, phlebotomists and surgeons, to name only a few. Because the nature of illness is often complex, care can involve a wide range of staff from the medical discipline working together. The intensive care team may need to work alongside orthopaedic surgeons, radiographers and nurses, for example. The ways in which these people work together is called inter-professional, as they work together within one profession but from the basis of different specialisms.

When thinking about supporting any one outcome for CYPF we may soon find that we need to consider involving a range of different professions from across disciplines. A young person who has been arrested will have come to the attention of the police; if they are in care they will also have a social worker; they could be at school and teachers may usefully be involved; they could have mental health issues and so CAMHS (Child and Adolescent Mental Health Service) could also support; and they could have been going to the same youth and community centre for years and feel like their youth worker has been their only constant adult. All these needs interact with one another in complex ways and cannot be separated out into neat boxes. In the same way, professionals who support CYPF cannot operate in silos, they need to interact. When different disciplines come together to support CYPF it is called multi-disciplinary or multi-agency working.

The main disciplines that support CYPF are considered to be education, policing, youth offending, social care, youth work and healthcare. Within each of these disciplines there may be many professionals involved – an arresting officer may work with a youth offending team for example. So inter-professional work can also occur alongside and within multi-agency work. Establishing this way of working was a focus of policy in the UK throughout the millennial decade due to the failure of multiple agencies to safeguard children who were being abused. The deaths of these individual children led to a policy for multi-agency work towards common outcomes (DfES, 2004; DfES, 2005) and tightened information sharing and communication protocols (Munro, 2011).

This introduces the inherent complexity in supporting wellbeing for CYPF, with potential differences of opinion between professionals within and between disciplines.

Wellbeing professionals

In many countries there is a dizzying number of professionals who contribute to the wellbeing of CYPF. In some countries, such as Finland and Northern Ireland, a holistic professional role has been created called a 'social pedagogue'. These practitioners are responsible for the holistic care of children over-coming some of the divides between education and care found elsewhere. However, these tend to be focused on the early years and as children grow into young people a range of disciplines will support wellbeing.

Table 2.1 shows a list of ten disciplines and associated professional roles that contribute to the wellbeing of CYPF.

This initial list includes more than titles, and there are many more missing. Each of the professionals in this list have had training within their discipline (e.g. criminal justice), and within their specialist role within that discipline (e.g. youth offending). Although all these professionals may contribute to wellbeing, they may all have a different perspective of what wellbeing is, and how they can best contribute to it. In the Introduction we established six different perspectives of wellbeing (see Table I.1), now we propose ten different disciplinary lenses to these nine perspectives of wellbeing.

To understand the ways in which professionals work with CYPF, and specifically wellbeing and social justice, we will investigate the 'construct' of the child, young person, or family, which they are working from.

Differing constructs of wellbeing

A construct is an idea or theory containing a range of concepts. For example, a construct of a child is a range of beliefs about the nature of children and childhood. As these beliefs are theoretical they are not necessarily 'the truth', although professionals may defend them as if they are true! The existence of

Table 2.1 Disciplines and professional roles in wellbeing

Discipline	Roles
Education	Adult and Community Education staff Further Education and College staff Teachers School Support staff Providers of extended activities Learning Mentors Behavioural and Educational Support Teams Inclusion Teams 14–19 Education providers Educational Psychologists Educational Welfare Officers Pastoral Support Workers School Library Service staff Workers in Cultural Heritage, Museums and Galleries Children's Centre staff Day Nursery staff Nursery School staff Registered Child Minders and Nannies Play Workers
Youth work	Youth Workers Youth Support Workers
Careers staff	Career Personal Advisers Job Centre Advisers
Housing	Young People's Housing and Accommodation Support Workers Youth Engagement Officers Community Development Officers
Sports	Sports Coaches Outdoor Education staff Health and Fitness staff Personal Trainers
Health	General Practitioners Primary and Community Health Practitioners Community Health Service staff Sexual Health Support Worker Drug and Alcohol Support Worker Mental Health Service staff Child and Adolescent Mental Health staff Health Visitors School Nurses Nurses Community Children's Nurses Paediatricians Psychiatrists Children's Allied Health Professionals Teenage Pregnancy Workers
Psychology	Educational Psychologists Community Psychologists

Justice	Youth Offending Teams Secure Training Centre staff Probation Officers Police and Law Enforcement Officers Community Safety Officers Prosecution Service staff Custodial Care Service staff Secure Unit staff
Social Care	Foster Carers Social Workers Registered Children's Homes staff Residential Childcare Workers Family Centre and Day Centre Workers Children and Family Court Advisory and Support Service Support Workers Portage Workers Child Support Agency staff Child Protection Officers Multi-agency Public Protection Teams Children's Services staff
Community development	Community Development Workers

varying constructs of the child itself demonstrates that there are multiple truths rather than a single one. Other complexities are at play when considering young people and the post-modernity conditions. This is extended further when considering the 'family' and challenges of understanding what constitutes family in modern society.

If we take children as a working example, professionals learn a particular version of the truth in training. Their discipline will have a certain construct of a child and childhood and this determines how they think about and work with children. Within each discipline, there will be training for different specialist roles, and this will further refine those professionals' views of the child, the goals of their work, and practice itself. The professional training, professional guidelines, codes of conduct and common accepted practices of the 60+ roles identified above, create an array of forms of practice (McKimm, 2009). Whilst this creates the rich diversity needed to support CYPF's needs, it also creates scope for disagreement as to what is the 'right' practice.

To exemplify this, we have deliberately chosen two professions with starkly different constructs and applied some crude generalisations; this is purely to emphasise our point rather than to contribute to stereotypes.

Traditionally and stereotypically youth workers' core belief is to value young people for who they are, regardless of what they do. They believe that young people can only be engaged on a voluntary basis, and work is built around the young person's interests alone. Youth workers' practice therefore involves supporting young people to explore who they are, what they want, and to help them to attain that within the parameters of the law.

Traditionally and stereotypically police officers' core belief is that justice needs to be upheld, and those who do not comply are punished or have their freedom restricted in order to uphold the law. From this perspective, young people who break the law need warnings, discipline, anti-social behaviour orders or imprisonment.

The youth workers' construct of childhood and youth is one of freedom and self-expression. The policing construct is of compliance to norms for the good of all. The potential difficulty of youth workers and police officers working together to decrease substance abuse is immediately apparent. Both sets of professionals perceive the same problem and they may attempt to solve it in very different ways. Neither of the approaches is right or wrong. The youth workers privilege the individual above society, and the police privilege society above the individual. Both can be seen to support wellbeing and social justice but in opposite ways.

These differing constructs will then influence which aspect of wellbeing is given more attention. It seems obvious, for example, that the health profession will view wellbeing as good health, but it is worth considering which aspects of wellbeing are naturally privileged by other sectors. These are identified in Table 2.2 below.

Table 2.2 Different professional constructs of the child and aspects of wellbeing focused on

Sector	Construct of the child	Aspect of wellbeing focused on
Education	Child learns and develops	Development of learning as wellbeing
Youth work	Child explores identity, can self-express and lives free from oppression, discrimination and marginalisation	Freedom from oppression as wellbeing
Careers staff	Child/young person enters employment	Employment status as wellbeing
Housing	Young person is able to be employed and become a good future tenant	Employment status and conformity to societal norms as wellbeing
Sports	Child is fit and healthy	Health wellbeing
Health	Child is healthy	Health wellbeing
Psychology	Child is psychologically well	Psychological wellbeing
Justice	Child conforms to societal laws	Absence of crime as wellbeing
Social Care	Child is safe and free from harm	Absence of harm as wellbeing
Community development	Child is included as an active part of a community	Social capital as wellbeing

These ten disciplinary perspectives on wellbeing can lead to confusion when the term 'wellbeing' is used uncritically. This is the difficulty with 'wellbeing' becoming a buzzword as its indiscriminate use and assumption of shared understanding breeds difficulties. For example, a team of practitioners may all agree to improve the wellbeing of a particular CYPF, but what they individually mean by that could lead to a variety of practices that they may not necessarily all agree to. This could lead to later conflict as divergent practices appear from what they thought was a common agreement.

The unveiling of the nine different perspectives of wellbeing in the introduction and ten disciplinary foci here cautions us against reductionism. Reductionism means reducing a complex term (wellbeing) to something simple and taken for granted. When we talk about wellbeing we need to be explicit about which aspect we are referring to rather than assuming a common frame of reference. We need to challenge ourselves to consider whether the constructs of CYPF and associated perspective on wellbeing is necessarily the most appropriate in any given circumstance, and consider how we can align disparate views.

Therefore our core argument to support work within these complexities entails some of the key concepts of critical pedagogy. In particular, critical dialogue is important here, so that we do not accept and take for granted, but problematise and make explicit our perspective and assumptions. This primarily includes assumptions about social justice and its relationship to wellbeing. This is the process of coming to shared broader aims.

Government and policy confusion

Not only is there potential for confusion and conflict between disciplines and specialist professional roles, but there is also confusion caused by the changing terms used by governments.

In the UK a political discourse based on 'need' developed into one of 'inclusion' and this has more recently changed to one of 'wellbeing'. But aren't having needs met and being included aspects of wellbeing – so is anything different meant by these changes in terminology? It is important to problematise, unpick and challenge what these terms mean politically, which aspects of wellbeing are emphasised, which are missing, and how the terminology services political purposes. In effect, the government in each country needs to be viewed as another 'discipline' with its own construct of CYPF. Where professional disciplines tend to have constructs that are fixed over time, the political construct can change dramatically in short spaces of time.

Practitioners need to navigate this changing policy context and make sense of the rhetoric of wellbeing in terms of their own practice values and methods. Again, criticality is needed in reading policy terms and what is meant between the lines.

Nick Axford from Dartington Social Research Unit (2008) simplified the different disciplinary constructs of wellbeing into five categories that focus on; need, rights, poverty, quality of life and social exclusion.

Axford concludes that through analysis of the constructs and the prevalence of associated issues in the UK's child population, all five views of wellbeing are useful and overlapping rather than discrete. He advocates for practitioners to see them in this way rather than treating a single perspective as their own preserve (2008: 183). As overlapping perspectives, the five categories and associated 'rich mix of services' create a framework to cohere practice. To understand what this rich mix might look like we will explore each category in a little more depth.

The perspective of **needs** seeks to address health and developmental impairments including education and behaviour both in terms of remedying current impairments and in terms of preventing impairments from developing from a risk assessment perspective.

The **rights** perspective sees wellbeing as the presence of the rights of the child, for example, to have protection, provision and participation as in the 1991 UN Convention on the Rights of the Child. Wellbeing initiatives here would focus on participation, advocacy and voice.

The **poverty** perspective sees wellbeing as having an adequate income and standard of living. Living in a household dependent on basic social assistance is seen as living in poverty. Provision here focuses on the alleviation of poverty.

The **quality of life** perspective seeks to improve CYPF objective circumstances and their subjective outlook on life. These combine into someone living 'a good life'. Quality of life is also enhanced with leisure opportunities and so wellbeing from this stance will seek to improve these.

Finally, the **social exclusion** perspective sees wellbeing as inclusion in mainstream society. This approach would seek to limit the social exclusion caused by disadvantages in education, employment or training, family, community and peer domains.

The strength of Axford's (2008) work is that the five terms encompass the objective, subjective, personal and social elements of wellbeing and all the disciplinary constructs listed earlier. Critically, however, the terminology is still opaque and many different interpretations could be read into them. The term 'quality of life', for example, could mean many things to many people.

This leads us to the key point of this chapter. The task that challenges us is not to find the right 'word' to define wellbeing, but rather to engage in meaningful dialogue with one another about what is meant by the terminology we use, so that all the professionals working with CYPF can support them coherently and in complementary ways.

Thriving not surviving

What may have become apparent in reading this chapter, is a discourse of 'enough' wellbeing and the accompanying practice of making up for things that are missing. This is a deficit discourse that identifies what is lacking, what is needed, and drives practice to compensate and address the need and the lacking.

The Positive Psychology movement takes great issue with this acceptance of 'good enough' wellbeing. For this movement, wellbeing goes beyond being OK and is about flourishing. From the flourishing perspective, Seligman (2011: 27) highlights the presence of five factors involved in wellbeing:

- Positive emotion
- Engagement
- Meaning
- Positive relationships
- Accomplishment

This list is very personal and subjective and stands in stark contrast to the national policies often aimed at alleviating poverty and obesity, for example. Positive Psychology sees wellbeing as more than meeting basic needs.

This aligns with Herzberg's (1966) model of motivation. Herzberg stated that certain basic conditions had to be in place in order to keep people motivated enough to come to work – these he called hygiene factors. Having put enough of these in place to address demotivation, the manager can then look to improve motivation. Herzberg identified a range of factors that made people pleased to be at work, these were called satisfiers and included setting your own goals, working autonomously and gaining promotion.

The parallel to wellbeing is that dominant practice focuses on the basic or hygiene factors of enabling CYPF to achieve a basic level of wellbeing by ensuring that there is nothing wrong. The challenge from Positive Psychology is for practice to also focus on ensuring there are good things in CYPF lives that enable them to flourish. Herzberg's model posits that basic needs have to be met before motivation can be increased. It is interesting to consider whether CYPF need basic wellbeing to be in place before they can flourish, or whether they can flourish despite a lack of wellbeing. That calls into question whether flourishing is an entirely psychological construct or one influenced by physical experience. What we consider important here is that CYPF are critically conscious and that this is the foundation of wellbeing. Awareness of what is, or could be, wrong, as well as what good things there are out there and how they access them are critical questions. We need to ensure our practice promotes these questions and provides safe spaces in which to explore the many complex answers they may provoke.

Increasingly the wide range of perspectives on wellbeing are brought together in holistic views and measures of wellbeing (Statham and Chase, 2010: 12–16). A challenge remains, however, in how that consensus is translated into practice. We believe that critical pedagogy answers this challenge. We position critical pedagogy as a multi-disciplinary and inter-professional practice that leads to increased wellbeing whether it is applied in a school, hospital, prison or street corner. This is the focus of this book from chapter four onwards, particularly through the use of case studies in part 2.

Professionals' wellbeing

Whilst focusing on the wellbeing of CYPF, we may ignore our own needs as practitioners. Over the last decade the field of employee wellbeing has developed, for both economic and humanistic reasons.

There has been a realisation in the last decade that absenteeism, presenteeism (employees at work but not working) and sickness costs organisations a huge amount of money and hinders their effectiveness and profitability. As a result a range of local, national and international projects have been launched that promote the resilience and wellbeing of employees. Whilst employees benefit personally from increased wellbeing, the driver of these projects is primarily the economic benefit derived by the organisations employing them.

In the UK these initiatives have been derived in part from annual data on workplace absence collected by the Chartered Institute of Personnel Development (CIPD, 2016). On average, UK employees are sick for 6.3 days a year with a median cost of £522 each. Absence was found to be markedly higher for employees in public services, who are away from work for 7.9 days each on average. We suspect that this trend might apply to all practitioners in high pressured helping services.

Business in the Community (BiC) (2013) claim that 20 million workers in the UK are not delivering to their full capability or are absent from work, costing the UK economy £17 billion year. They also found that only 40% of employees trust their employer. As a result BiC (2013) have created a set of international standards to allow organisations to publicly report on their employee engagement and wellbeing. This information, they state, is key to organisational productivity and therefore of prime interest to investors and other stakeholders.

Case studies are emerging of individual organisations which are working hard to improve the wellbeing of their employees now that the economic value of this has been realised. The most notable of these is Unilever which has developed a four-pillar programme to boost physical and mental wellbeing. The four pillars are:

- Leader and manager awareness of issues and how to deal with them through training
- A culture of communication supported by tools and continuous reinforcement
- Preventative tools to help individuals avoid issues
- Organisational support when issues occur (CIPD, 2014: 29–30).

When large corporates such as Unilever champion wellbeing, other organisations, agencies and governments take note.

It is important that the professionals who are responsible for the wellbeing of CYPF experience wellbeing themselves. Yet they are often working in difficult environments, with a lack of organisational stability, few resources, and little time. Measures such as supervision and approaches such as reflective practice are inconsistent across disciplines. With this in mind, the vignette below highlights the recent NHS workplace wellbeing charter, which could usefully be applied to all organisations that work with CYPF.

Vignette 2.1 The NHS Workplace Wellbeing Charter

According to the Office of National Statistics 131 million days were lost due to sickness absences in the UK in 2013 (NHS, 2014). The cost of sickness and absence has led the NHS to create standards for wellbeing in the UK. There are three levels of engagement with the charter:

- **Level one:** Commitment to meeting the basic level of all standards
- **Level two:** Achieve by actively encouraging positive lifestyle choices and addressing health issues
- **Level three:** Fully engaged leadership with a range of programmes and support mechanisms

Within each of the three levels there are standards to address leadership, culture and communication. There is an online self-assessment tool, a toolkit, and a formal assessment by independent consultants to grant the achievement of excellence standards and national recognition as an organisation that promotes employee wellbeing.

Although the standards are voluntary rather than statutory, their publication and endorsement by the NHS adds legitimacy to the work of agencies such as BiC and individual organisations such as Unilever.

Whilst the NHS does genuinely want to support the wellbeing of all members of the UK public, some of the motivation for the charter may be the potential cost savings to the NHS created by employers supporting employee wellbeing.

Reflective activity

Do you think you are surviving or thriving in your practice?

Is there room within your practice to be reflective and consider the relationship between your wellbeing and your practice?

Do you have opportunities to discuss your practice in formal settings such as supervision, team reviews or action learning sets?

Summary of key points

We have demonstrated that there are different views of how to support the 'wellbeing' of CYPF due to the different constructs of childhood and wellbeing held by disciplines and professionals.

We have explored some of the challenges of aligning practice holistically and highlighted that dialogue is needed to unpack the meaning of our everyday language. We also introduced the notion that a basic level of wellbeing could be a limiting goal, and that practice should perhaps aim to enable CYPF to flourish.

We put forward the argument, that in order to work within these complexities entails some of the key concepts of critical pedagogy. Critical dialogue ensures that we do not accept and take for granted, but problematise and make explicit our perspective and assumptions. This primarily includes assumptions about social justice and its relationship to wellbeing. This is the process of coming to shared broader aims. The task that challenges us is not to find the right 'word' to define wellbeing, but rather to engage in meaningful dialogue with one another about what is meant by the terminology we use, so that all the professionals working with CYPF can support them coherently and in complementary ways.

To conclude, we highlight the need for the professionals who work with CYPF to experience wellbeing themselves.

Further reading

Aked, J., Marks, N., Cordon, C., and Thompson, S. (2008). *Five Ways to Wellbeing: The Evidence*. London: nef.

Axford, N. (2008). *Exploring Concepts of Child Wellbeing*. London: Polity Press.

Children's Society (2014). *The Good Childhood Report*. London: Children's Society.

Rees, G., and Main, G. (eds) (2015). *Children's Views on Their Lives and Well-being in 15 countries: An Initial Report on the Children's Worlds Survey, 2013–14*. York, UK: Children's Worlds Project (ISCWeB).

References

Axford, N. (2008). *Exploring Concepts of Child Well-Being. Implications for Children's Services*. Bristol: Policy Press.

Business in the Community (BiC) (2013). *Workwell: BITC Public Reporting Guidelines. Employee Engagement and Wellbeing*. London: BITC.

CIPD (2014). *Absence Management 2014*. London: CIPD and Simply Health.

CIPD (2016). *Absence Management 2016*. London: CIPD and Simply Health.

Department for Education and Skills (DfES) (2004). *Every Child Matters: Change for Children*. London: DfES.

Department for Education and Skills (DfES) (2005). *Youth Matters. Cm 6629*. London: HMSO.

Herzberg, Frederick (1966). *Work and the Nature of Man*. Cleveland: World Publishing.

McKimm, J. (2009). 'Professional Roles and Workforce Development', in McKimm, J. and Phillips, K. (eds.) *Leadership and Management of Integrated Services.* Poole: Learning Matters, pp. 122–140.

Munro (2011). 'The Munro review of child protection: final report, a child-centred system CM, 8062'. The Stationery Office, London, UK.

NHS (2014). *The Workplace Wellbeing Charter: National Award for England.* Liverpool: Liverpool City Council Health at Work and NHS England.

Seligman, M. (2011). *Flourish: A New Understanding of Happiness and Wellbeing and How to Achieve Them.* London: Nicholas Brearley.

Statham, J., and Chase, E. (2010). *Childhood Wellbeing: A Brief Introduction.* London: The Childhood Wellbeing Research Centre.

3 Wellbeing from global perspectives

Chapter overview:

We wanted to write this book grounded in practice and our experience of practice is within the UK. Therefore, it is critical to situate this practice within wider global perspectives. The global perspective contextualises wellbeing, as well as drawing in learning from wider perspectives, for the reader to bring to their understanding. Wellbeing is an international phenomenon, and arguably no one nation can work on it in isolation from the wider world. This chapter explores the global development perspective overarching international wellbeing. The chapter then progresses to analyse a variety of wellbeing policies and associated measures. The evidence for a lack of social justice within and between countries is revealed through a comparison of global measures of wellbeing.

Global development and economics

Economic measures were historically used to demonstrate the 'progress' or 'development' that a country makes. The more uniform these economic measures, the easier it was to compare relative levels of international development. The assumption behind the economic measures of development is that the more money a country has, the greater their productivity and economic growth, and therefore the more 'well' people would be. In crude terms, this associates wealth with wellbeing.

A renaissance in thinking about global development was led by Sen (1999) who redefined development as freedom. Other contributors to this renaissance were Wilkinson and Pickett (2010) who demonstrated that material wealth did not equate to wellbeing. Sen eloquently introduces his concept of development as inverse freedom. A lack of development is evidenced by the 'unfreedoms' of poverty, poor economic conditions, deprivation, lack of public facilities, intolerance and oppression. These 'unfreedoms' go beyond pure economic measures and are as applicable to modern world countries as their, so-called, third world cousins. Freedom is therefore the key to development, as Sen (1999: 11) states, "With adequate social opportunities, individuals can effectively shape their own destiny and help each other". This obviously chimes with the social justice interface with wellbeing that we are advocating within this book.

This focus drives countries to create more personal, social and economic freedom, rather than have more economic wealth. If more people in the country have more freedom across these domains, then more of them will experience social justice and wellbeing. Development as freedom is the economics of social justice. The increase of freedoms created then serves as a measure of the development of a country (Sen, 1999: 4), and so freedom is both the means and end of development (ibid: 36).

In *The Spirit Level*, Wilkinson and Pickett (2010: 4) startled the world with their stark proof that economic growth did not contribute to social wellbeing. Their argument, like Sen's, is focused on the need for increased social justice.

Just one of Wilkinson and Pickett's compelling analyses shows that as countries get wealthier, the relationship with life expectancy weakens. Their data shows that whilst poverty is associated to poor life expectancy because of a lack of basic nutrition, or incorrect nutrition, wealth is associated with poor life expectancy because of cardiovascular disease and high blood pressure. These are the ailments of affluence and over-indulgence! Whilst the wealthier live longer than the poor, in absolute terms, there is a tipping point at which increased money no longer leads to increased longevity. Money does not have a linear relationship with health wellbeing.

Wilkinson and Pickett's analyses span poverty, mental health, drug use, life expectancy, obesity, educational performance, teenage births, violence, imprisonment and social mobility. As they conclude:

> We have seen that the rich countries have got to the end of the really important contributions which economic growth can make to the quality of life and also that our future lies in improving the quality of the social environments in our societies. The role of this book is to point out that greater equality is the material foundation on which better social relations are built (2010: 272).

The reason we introduce this perspective within this chapter, rather than earlier, is its relationship with relative concepts of wealth internationally. The relative wellbeing of all inhabitants of a country, and of the globe, is important. Development is contingent on everyone being well. This perspective has had impact on the behaviour of politicians and development agencies worldwide. For example, Alsop and Heinsohn (2005: 5) state, "Empowerment is now found in the documentation of over 1800 World Bank aided projects and it is the subject of debate and analytic work within the development community". Further, many countries are now embedding wellbeing into policy frameworks.

However, there is important questioning to be made of whether the introduction of wellbeing measures is placatory practice, designed to reassure and quieten the dissenters, rather than truly tackling the deeply ingrained financial imperatives behind a lot of governmental thinking. Recent recessions in the UK have triggered a policy and media insistence on the market economy as the only form of recovery. This raises concerns about how seriously governments take wellbeing compared to cash.

Vignette 3.1 The New Zealand Wellbeing Policy

Dalziel and Saunders (2015: 12) propose a wellbeing policy for New Zealand that synthesises the work of proponents of the economics of wellbeing. The framework is based on five principles:

Principle 1: The purpose of economic activity is to promote the wellbeing of persons.

Principle 2: The wellbeing of persons is related to their capabilities to lead the kinds of lives they value and have reason to value.

Principle 3: Economic policies should expand the substantive freedom of persons to lead the kinds of lives they value and have reason to value.

Principle 4: Wellbeing is created through persons making time-use choices they judge will contribute to their leading the kinds of lives they value.

Principle 5: Market production should enable persons to add value to the kinds of lives they value.

A range of measures are identified by the authors that already allow the capture of relevant data, including:

- New Zealand Time Use Survey
- Child Poverty Monitor
- New Zealand Values Survey
- Statistics New Zealand
- Household Economic Survey.

The authors state that:

> there is an opportunity for New Zealand to pioneer ... a shift from a 'welfare state' to a 'wellbeing state'. The fundamental difference is where agency is thought to lie: in a welfare state, it is accepted that agency lies primarily with central government and the public service; in a wellbeing state, agency is conceived as lying primarily with the country's citizens.

Whilst the New Zealand Government may not have embraced this wellbeing policy framework wholesale, some of the principles are recognisable in the Better Public Services programme (Wevers, 2011; Ryan, 2012) and Treasury's Living Standards Framework (Gleisner *et al.*, 2011; Gleisner *et al.*, 2012; Karacaoglu, 2012).

As a consequence of the link between wellbeing and progress, measuring wellbeing has become a common phenomenon in contemporary times. As finance is a common unit of measure that can be exchanged between countries, it has also been the prime unit of measure. A new trend has emerged, however, led by Amartya Sen that sees development from a broader perspective. When wellbeing is seen holistically, then measures of wellbeing will offer a view of how society is developing in the round, rather than focusing on economic measures as proxies for wellbeing. This message was reinforced in 2005 with the Organisation for Economic Co-operation and Development (OECD) World Forum declaration of the need for international data on wellbeing. This was further reinforced in 2009 with the European Commission paper 'Beyond GDP' calling for better measures of human wellbeing across Europe. In the same year the Commission on the Measurement of Economic Performance and Social Progress called for international measures of GDP, quality of life and sustainability. As a direct result of these international economic drivers, there is now a range of comparative data available on wellbeing.

International comparisons of wellbeing

There is a wide range of comparisons of wellbeing between countries. The research varies in terms of the range of countries included, the definition of wellbeing applied, who is involved and the tools or indicators used to measure that version of wellbeing. Statistical comparisons of global wellbeing therefore need to be read critically. The rankings or percentile scores are meaningless without an understanding of where they were collected, with whom, by whom, with what purpose and using which tools.

As a result, the different comparisons cannot be compared themselves, unless they are repeated with exactly the same parameters year on year. The most informative measures are therefore those that have been repeated year on year in the same way. They are starting to reveal trends in wellbeing.

As we live in the UK we have identified the position of the UK in a range of comparative data sets. This was done for illustrative purposes to allow you to see the variety of rankings of one country across different measures, and also to highlight that although a first world country, the UK does not fare well in terms of wellbeing. This is exemplified in Table 3.1, with some examples detailed further below.

The 2012 UNICEF report 11

The purpose of the UNICEF Report Card series is: "to encourage the monitoring of children's well-being, to permit country comparisons, and to stimulate debate and the development of policies to improve children's lives" (Adamson, 2012: 1). The concept of child wellbeing used in this measure is guided by the UN Convention on the Rights of the Child. In 2007 you will note the UK at

Table 3.1 The UK's ranking in international comparisons of wellbeing

2007 UNICEF report 7	21st out of 21
2009 OECD report	28th out of 30
2009 European Index	24th out of 29
2012 UNICEF report 11	16th out of 29
2014 Good Childhood Report	31st out of 39
2015 Children's Worlds Survey	14th out of 15

the bottom of the league table in Report Card 7. By 2012 the UK's position has improved in relative terms with a ranking of 16th out of 29 in Report Card 11. Whilst this measure is apparently the same, the number of countries has leapt from 21 to 29. This makes it impossible to determine whether the UK has improved or not. If the countries newly included had very poor wellbeing then the UK would advance in the rankings with no improvement in the UK, and conversely if the new countries all had good to excellent wellbeing then the UK must have done a lot in the five years to have improved its ranking. Issues therefore remain in taking data at face value.

The UNICEF report measures wellbeing across the following five areas:

Material well-being – monetary deprivation (relative child poverty rate; relative child poverty gap); material deprivation (deprivation index; low family affluence rate)

Health – health at birth (infant mortality rate; low birth weight rate); preventive health (immunisation rate); childhood mortality (ages 1–19)

Education – participation rate in early childhood education; further education (15–19 years old); numbers of 15–19 year olds not in education, employment or training (NEET); achievement (average PISA scores in reading, maths and science)

Behaviour and risks – health behaviours (overweight, eating fruit, eating breakfast, taking exercise); risk behaviours (teenage pregnancy rate, smoking, alcohol, drugs); exposure to violence (bullying, fighting)

Housing and environment – housing (persons per room, multiple housing problems); environmental safety (homicide rate, air pollution) (2012, 2).

Despite the concerns expressed above, the data does allow UNICEF to identify important trends. For example, overall, between 2000–01 and 2009–10, there was widespread improvement in most, if not all, indicators of children's wellbeing. This was particularly the case for family affluence, infant mortality and smoking among children. The potential of this UNICEF report to shame individual countries has perhaps spurred them all on, and these overall statistical changes perhaps demonstrate international efforts to better support basic needs. The report therefore has an important role in global development.

Interestingly the Netherlands has so far retained its position as leader of wellbeing rankings. It was the only country ranked among the top five in all dimensions of child wellbeing which must prompt international interest in how they achieve this. Four other Nordic countries (Finland, Iceland, Norway and Sweden) also ranked just below the Netherlands at the top of the table showing an interesting geographic or political trend in Scandinavia.

The bottom four places in the table were occupied by three of the poorest countries in the survey (Latvia, Lithuania and Romania) accompanied, contentiously, by the United States, one of the richest. From this, UNICEF conclude that, "there does not appear to be a strong relationship between per capita GDP and overall child well-being – in other words, country wealth does not always mean happier and healthier children. But investment in children is important" (2012, 3). This supports the views of Sen and Wilkinson and Pickett discussed earlier.

Unpacking the UK-specific results raises interesting questions too. 86% of UK children reported a high level of life satisfaction. But which children were asked, who asked them, how were they asked, and how socially just was this process? The UK's child mortality rate of 4.4 mortalities per 1000 live births is approximately double the rate of Sweden or Finland. Which children are dying? Of what causes? Under what circumstances? What are Sweden and Finland doing differently?

The UK has the lowest further education participation rate in the developed world at 74 per cent and almost 10 per cent of young people are not in education, employment or training. Why are our schools and colleges failing children? Why is education not valuable to young people in the UK?

The UK ranks 27th out of 29 countries for teenage pregnancy rates. How many of the teenage pregnancies are positive choices to parent? How many teenage mums thrive with a new-born child?

The value of these reports also lies in the critical questions that arise from the detailed results for each country. Each indicator reveals issues with far ranging policy implications. It would be fantastic for governments to focus on wellbeing as an intrinsically good thing, but it is also a good thing if these 'league tables' are embarrassing them into tackling wellbeing.

The Children's Worlds Report (Reece and Main, 2015)

This report took an entirely subjective stance and ranked 15 countries according to the views of 30,000 children aged 10–12. A survey was administered across the 15 countries and there were three versions of the questionnaire for the different age groups – for children around 8, 10 and 12 years of age respectively. These collected details of:

- Basic characteristics (age, gender, country of birth)
- Living situation, home and family relationships
- Money and economic circumstances

- Friends and other relationships
- Local area
- School
- Time use
- Self
- Overall subjective wellbeing
- Children's rights (2015: 14).

The mean scores in 2015 showed significant variations by indicator and country. For example:

- Romania scores highly on all indicators and Colombia and Turkey do so on most of them.
- South Korea scores low on all indicators and the UK and South Africa score low for all but one indicator each
- Some countries show greater fluctuations in ranking
- Algeria is ranked in the top three countries for family life and life as a student but in the bottom three countries for material possessions and friends
- Germany is in the top three countries for friends but in the bottom three for life as a student and local area (2015: 133).

Focusing this in on the UK, the report shows that 8–12 year olds in the UK do not think they experience wellbeing across a comprehensive range of measures and ranked 14th out of 15. Despite the perceived development within and desirability of the UK (evidenced by recent trends in immigration), children in the UK do not experience wellbeing. This raises questions as to whether this lack of wellbeing is perceptual or if it correlates to objective wellbeing? We also need to question which 30,000 children completed it, with whom, and how. Further consideration needs to be given to how a perceived lack of wellbeing can be addressed.

The European Personal and Social Wellbeing Survey (2015)

This index attempts to measure multidimensional wellbeing. In order to do this there is a comprehensive range of indicators clustered into six areas of wellbeing. These are shown in Table 3.2 below.

The combination of personal and social wellbeing and objective and subjective wellbeing is evident within the survey items. The survey found that whilst the overall evaluative wellbeing score was often a predictor of scores in all categories, this was not always the case. Some of the dimensions behaved differently in different countries. This, the authors state, supports the view that wellbeing is both a multi-dimensional concept, and culturally sensitive (ESS, 2015: 7).

Table 3.2 The UK's ranking in international comparisons of wellbeing

Wellbeing Survey Item	ESS Survey Item
Evaluative wellbeing	How satisfied with life as a whole How happy I am
Emotional wellbeing	Felt sad, how often last week Felt depressed, how often last week Enjoyed life, how often last week Were happy, how often last week Felt anxious, how often last week Felt calm and peaceful, how often last week
Functioning	Free to decide how to live my life Little chance to show how capable I am Feel accomplishment from what I do Interested in what I am doing Enthusiastic about what I am doing Feel what I do in life is valuable and worthwhile Have a sense of direction Always optimistic about my future There are lots of things I feel I am good at In general feel very positive about myself At times feel as if I am a failure When things go wrong in my life it takes me a long time to get back to normal Deal with important problems
Vitality	Felt everything I did was an effort, how often past week Sleep was restless, how often past week Could not get going, how often past week Had lot of energy, how often past week
Community wellbeing	Most people can be trusted/can't be too careful People try to take advantage Most of the time people are helpful Feel people in local area are a help to one another Feel close to the people in the local area
Supportive relationships	How many with whom I can discuss intimate issues Feel appreciated by those I am close to Receive help and support Felt lonely, how often past week

Other pollsters (e.g. Gallup, 2015) seem to ignore these cultural sensitivities and the multi-dimensional nature of wellbeing, and confidently publish league tables of countries' levels of thriving, struggling and surviving, which are subjective concepts in their own right. The results are based on interviews with only 1000 people in each country over a five-year span. The scale of the research is too small and the duration too long for them to be robust and representative of wellbeing internationally.

The key message here is that we must all have our wits about us when engaging with the research and findings on international wellbeing.

Vignette 3.2 How the UK measures wellbeing

The UK's Office of National Statistics (ONS, 2015) was tasked with measuring wellbeing in the UK. The measures are diverse and attempt to incorporate many aspects of wellbeing. They state that within the UK, there is a commitment to developing wider measures of wellbeing so that government policies can be more tailored to the things that matter. Wider and systematic consideration of wellbeing has the potential to lead to better decisions by government, markets and the public and, as such, better outcomes.

Wellbeing in the UK is measured across ten different domains with between three and six indicators each as shown in Table 3.3 below.

Table 3.3 UK National Wellbeing Indicators

Personal wellbeing	1.1	Very high rating of satisfaction with their lives overall
	1.2	Very high rating of how worthwhile the things they do are
	1.3	Rated their happiness yesterday as very high
	1.4	Rated their anxiety yesterday as very low
	1.5	Population mental wellbeing
Our relationships	2.1	Average rating of satisfaction with family life
	2.2	Average rating of satisfaction with social life
	2.3	Has spouse, family member or friend to rely on if they have a serious problem
Health	3.1	Healthy life expectancy at birth
	3.2	Reported long-term illness and a disability
	3.3	Somewhat, mostly or completely satisfied with their health
	3.4	Some evidence indicating depression or anxiety
What we do	4.1	Unemployment rate
	4.2	Somewhat, mostly or completely satisfied with their job
	4.3	Somewhat, mostly or completely satisfied with their amount of leisure time
	4.4	Volunteered more than once in the last 12 months
	4.5	Engaged with or participated in arts or cultural activity at least three times in last year
	4.6	Adult participation in 30 minutes of moderate intensity of sport, once per week

Where we live	5.1	Crimes against the person (per 1000 adults)
	5.2	Felt fairly/very safe walking alone after dark
	5.3	Accessed natural environment at least once a week in the last 12 months
	5.4	Agreed/agreed strongly they felt they belonged to their neighbourhood
	5.5	Households with good transport access to key services or work
	5.6	Fairly/very satisfied with their accommodation
Personal finance	6.1	Individuals in households with less than 60% of median income after housing costs
	6.2	Median wealth per household, including pension wealth
	6.3	Real median household income
	6.4	Somewhat, mostly or completely satisfied with the income of their household
	6.5	Report finding it quite or very difficult to get by financially
The economy	7.1	Real net national disposable income per head
	7.2	UK public sector net debt as a percentage of Gross Domestic Product
	7.3	Inflation rate
Education and skills	8.1	Human capital – the value of individuals' skills, knowledge and competencies in the labour market
	8.2	Five or more GCSEs A* to C including English and Maths
	8.3	UK residents aged 16–64 with no qualifications
Governance	9.1	Voter turnout in General Elections
	9.2	Those who have trust in national government
The natural environment	10.1	Total greenhouse gas emissions
	10.2	Protected areas in the UK (million hectares)
	10.3	Energy consumed within the UK from renewable sources
	10.4	Household waste that is recycled

The framework is to be commended as largely jargon free, and wide reaching across personal and social, objective and subjective indicators. Much data is already captured by statutory organisations and fed to the ONS, capitalising on existing data. For example, schools have a statutory duty to make annual returns to enable government to monitor school performance. This data corpus is used again in the wellbeing measure allowing analysis of levels of education and skills. Some of the indicators are new, however, and as a result have been added into national census activities such as the Annual Population Survey (ONS, 2014) which involves around 300,000 people in the UK. However, again we have to wonder which families are most likely to complete those surveys and if this is representative?

Data has been collected three times and the annual comparisons produce the following headlines:

Compared with a year earlier, 33% of indicators had improved, 42% showed no overall change, 21% were not assessed and 5% deteriorated (health satisfaction, anxiety or depression, satisfaction with leisure time, sense of safety for females at night, real median household income, satisfaction with household income, human capital, voter turnout).

The proportion of people in the UK giving the highest ratings for each aspect of personal wellbeing increased significantly in the financial year ending 2014.

Healthy life expectancy in the UK improved between 2006 to 2008 and 2009 to 2011, while the proportion of people satisfied with their health in the financial year ending 2013 showed no overall change.

Adult participation in 30 minutes of moderate intensity sport at least once a week in the UK improved over 3 years between 2010 to 2011 and 2013 to 2014, but deteriorated compared with 2012 to 2013.

In the financial year ending 2013, 21% of people in the UK lived in households with less than 60% of median income.

In the financial year ending 2013, 10.1% of people found it difficult to get by financially in the UK, an improvement since the financial years ending 2012 (10.9%) and 2010 (12.3%).

(ONS, 2015: 2).

There are many important questions that arise from these findings. In particular:

What accounts for these results? There is no mechanism for understanding what has led to change or stasis and there is no attribution, which is a serious limitation to the survey. Without this understanding it is hard to ascertain what to do to further improve wellbeing.

The second question is whether this data has had any impact on policy or practice, or it simply remains an interesting data set. This is the most significant challenge for any country – far greater than that of collating the data in the first place.

Despite these drawbacks and concerns that the measures are placatory, it is heartening to see that data has been collected and interrogated. This is at least creating the potential for change and increased social justice.

The happiness debate

Some academics believe that happiness is a better measure of wellbeing than the indicators suggested to date (Helliwell, Layard and Sachs, 2015). They advocate that perceived happiness should be the acid test for the efficacy of any policy. They propose a cost benefit analysis of the additional happiness bought per dollar of expenditure on a project. As a result, a UK based think tank called the New Economics Foundation (nef) produced an annual Happy Planet Index.

The index has an important contribution to make to our understanding of the measurement of wellbeing. The index is calculated from multiplying life satisfaction data from the Gallup World Poll with life expectancy data from United Nations and inequality data (the distribution of longevity and happiness outcomes in each country). This is then divided by the ecological footprint of each country, taken from the Global Footprint Network data. Several observations can be made from this. Firstly, this is another example of researchers drawing on existing data sets rather than reinvesting in more data collection. Secondly, it has a measure of social justice embedded within it. The use of measures of inequality data in an overall index is an important development supporting social justice. Thirdly, this measure also considers ecological concerns that have gone beyond the scope of other measures (and the scope of this book).

However, whilst the measure has undoubtedly progressed the measurement of social justice, its key conceptual term 'happiness' has come under sharp critique. 'Happiness' can be even more subjective than wellbeing. How individuals feel happy, why and when is incredibly variable. I, for example, feel very happy climbing a steep rock face, whilst another person would be very unhappy in the same situation. This highly contextually contingent nature of happiness has led to academics saying it is not possible to measure it reliably (Stewart, 2014). Perhaps this is why the Happy Planet Index does not directly measure 'happiness'. The closest it comes is using existing measures of quality of life, which is much less contentious. The 'happy' part of this index would therefore seem to be philosophically rather than methodologically aligned with Layard's happiness movement.

The third Happy Planet report written in 2012 (Murphy, 2012) showed that we are still living in an unhappy world. The report states it can "confirm that we are still not living on a happy planet, with no country achieving high and sustainable well-being and only nine close to doing so" (2012: 3). Interestingly, eight of those nine countries are in Latin America and the Caribbean, and the scores of high-income countries are brought down considerably by their large ecological footprints. This is exemplified by the US ranking 105th out of 151 countries. The addition of inequality outcomes and ecological footprint radically changes rankings, and will hopefully provoke further debate and change internationally.

Reflective activity

How do international comparisons support you to work on wellbeing in your own country?

How effective are your national measures of wellbeing?

How does your own work to support wellbeing compare to national and international measures?

Write a list of indicators that you could use to track the wellbeing of the people you work with year on year.

Summary of key points

Through this chapter we have demonstrated that wellbeing has now become synonymous with development, rather than wealth. Development is discussed in terms of freedom and unfreedom, which are characterised beyond pure economic measures. This perspective aligns with the relationship between social justice and wellbeing, inasmuch as freedom is the key to development and thus wellbeing and thus creating opportunities for personal, social and economic freedom are essential. This is equally applicable in both developed and developing countries.

Due to this, many countries now measure wellbeing. International comparisons are emphasising the importance of wellbeing and compelling governments worldwide to be attentive to it. Interesting results have emerged, further emphasising that wealth is not the key defining factor in wellbeing. Questions remain about the interventions and measurement that have an impact positively or adversely on wellbeing at a national and international level. We must pay attention to this questioning in our assumptions and draw from global perspectives in developing our practice.

Further reading

ONS (2015). *Measuring National Well-being: Life in the UK 2015*. London: ONS.
Sen, A. (1999). *Development as Freedom*. Oxford: Oxford University Press.
Wilkinson, R., and Pickett, K. (2010). *The Spirit Level: Why Equality is Better for Everyone*. London: Penguin.

References

Adamson, P. (2012). *Measuring Child Poverty, No. 10*. Florence: UNICEF Innocenti Report Centre.
Alsop, R., and Heinsohn, N. (2005). *Measuring Empowerment in Practice: Structuring Analysis and Framing Indicators. World Bank Research Working Paper*. World Bank.
Dalziel, P., and Saunders, C. (2015). 'Wellbeing Economics: A Policy Framework for New Zealand', *New Zealand Sociology*, 30(3), 8–26.

ESS (2015). *European's Personal and Social Wellbeing. Results from round 6 of the European Social Survey.* London: ESS.

Gallup (2015). *Gallup Global Wellbeing.* Washington: Gallup.

Gleisner, B., Llewellyn-Fowler, M., and McAlister, F. (2011). *Working Towards Higher Living Standards for New Zealanders.* Wellington: New Zealand Treasury, available at www.treasury.govt.nz/abouttreasury/higherlivingstandards

Gleisner, B., McAlister, F., Galt, M. and Beaglehole, J. (2012). 'A Living Standards Approach to Public Policy Making', *New Zealand Economic Papers*, 46(3), 211–238.

Helliwell, J., Layard, R., and Sachs, J. (2015). *The World Happiness Report 2015.* New York: Sustainable Development Solutions Network.

Karacaoglu, G. (2012) 'Improving the Living Standards of New Zealanders: Moving from a Framework to Implementation.' Presentation to the Wellbeing and Public Policy conference, Victoria University of Wellington, 13–15 June, available at www.treasury.govt.nz/abouttreasury/higherlivingstandards

Murphy, M., (2012) *The Happy Planet Index: 2012 Report: A Global Index of Sustainable Well-being.* London: nef.

Organisation for Economic Co-operation and Development (OECD) (2009). *World Forum Statistics, Knowledge and Policy Proceedings.* Paris: OECD.

ONS (2014). *Personal Wellbeing Survey User Guide (2013–14) Dataset.* London: ONS.

ONS (2015). *Measuring National Well-being: Life in the UK 2015.* London: ONS.

Reece, G. and Main, G. (eds) (2015). *Children's Views on their Lives and Well-being in 15 Countries: An Initial Report on the Children's Worlds Survey, 201--14.* York, UK: Children's Worlds Project (ISCWeB).

Ryan, B. (2012). 'Better Public Services a Window of Opportunity', *Public Services Quarterly*, 8(3), 1–25.

Sen, A. (1999). *Development as Freedom.* Oxford: Oxford University Press.

Stewart, F. (2014). 'Against Happiness: A Critical Appraisal of the Use of Measures Of Happiness for Evaluating Progress in Development', *Journal of Human Development and Capabilities: A Multi-Disciplinary Journal for People-Centered Development*, 15(4), 293–307.

Wevers, M. (2011). *Better Public Services.* Auckland: New Zealand Advisory Group for Better Public Services.

Wilkinson, R., and Pickett, K. (2010). *The Spirit Level: Why Equality is Better for Everyone.* London: Penguin.

4 Wellbeing and critical pedagogy

Chapter overview

Chapter 1 introduced the relationship between wellbeing and social justice. We showed how the two concepts are inextricably linked and mutually reinforcing. When we consider wellbeing in this way, we are looking at it through a particular lens. This forms the approach which we can take as practitioners to supporting CYPF wellbeing and social justice. Our approach is also described as our pedagogy; that is, the art or science of our teaching or facilitation of education, growth or change. Critical pedagogy is the approach which we take to achieving social justice and therefore, in this context, wellbeing. Through this chapter we propose a critical pedagogy for practice that supports CYPF wellbeing and social justice.

It is important to have a good understanding of what underpins critical pedagogy if we are to justify this as our approach to practice. We aim to do this by guiding you through the roots and history of critical pedagogy via key theorists and core theories.

What is critical pedagogy?

It may be a surprise for some, but not for many of us, to hear that there are different ways of learning and thus educating. There are clearly dominant approaches, but these should not be confused as the only way. Our discussion here is of CYPF wellbeing and social justice, how this is achieved in the world and our role as facilitators of this. Therefore this discussion is not constrained to schooling; it is concerned with learning, growth, development, transformation and emancipation. It is concerned with how we can facilitate this process.

Our pedagogy is our approach to this; our philosophy, our thinking, our theory and our practice of education. Once this is established we can consider where this takes place, but again, this is not limited to school. Learning happens everywhere, so what is our role in supporting this and creating more specific contexts and conditions of facilitating and drawing out learning?

Dewey (1963) referred to this as a social process. It is how CYPF engage with the world. Further it is how they understand the world; understand their place in the world and how they act in the world.

This particular approach to considering our facilitation of learning asks CYPF to discover the world, not just accept it as it is presented to them or how they find themselves in it. It encourages exploration, challenge and questioning. Thus, as facilitators of this approach to learning, how do we go about this, when other, more traditional and more dominant approaches are *telling* CYPF what to know, or how life is, as well as how and where to know it?

This perspective is essential when considering CYPF wellbeing and social justice. We cannot tell CYPF to be well; that they are feeling good; to memorise the equation of flourishing and that this will equate to them immediately flourishing; or that they are this percentage of resilient. Equally, we cannot pour equitable facts into their heads and expect them to come out the other side with rights, fairness and wealth.

This is not to entirely discredit other approaches to education, which critical pedagogy challenges in its justification of itself. There are times when factual dissemination is important and memorising of formulas is significant. A critical approach to learning is interested in broader, more overarching concerns, such as wellbeing and social justice, which facilitate CYPF through awareness of the world – its injustices and justices, their rights to access, and their functioning in the world. This engages CYPF in a different way – they learn what they want to learn, how they learn it and when they want to learn it. It becomes an exploration where they seek knowledge, rather than having knowledge done to them. At this point, we argue, CYPF are more likely to be ready to receive types of factual knowledge, previously 'done to' them. They might seek this out from educators or services who hold particular facts that will help them learn and grow. They have an intrinsic understanding of who they are, what they are interested in knowing and want to go out in search of it.

As workers, we are not only a facilitator at this point, we are a resource for CYPF to tap into. The science teacher and classroom become someone and somewhere young people want to engage with to seek knowledge; the youth worker is someone who listens and helps them realise that they are in an exploitative relationship, rather than telling the young person "he's not good for you"; the social worker becomes a caring support mechanism of safety and signposting, rather than the person who will split your family up.

A critical approach to this type of learning and knowing places the worker's emphasis on facilitating awareness, leading to embodied engagement, consideration, understanding and transformation. Therefore, as workers we are concerned with how we facilitate truly transformative learning that is concerned with the whole person, not just the cognitive, not just memorised facts, but CYPF knowing and feeling their place in the world; knowing and feeling well in the world; functioning and flourishing in the world.

For Ledwith (2005), this involves questioning, naming, reflecting, analysing, and acting that liberates people and communities. Traditional education has perhaps neglected this emancipatory aim and edge of criticality. Ledwith states, "People make critical connections when they link culture, political, social and economic issues with their everyday life experience. This counters the apathy and passivity symptomatic of a culture of silence" (2005: 59).

Critical pedagogy has a long history and wide range of contributing theories and theorists. These have defined the focus, content and style of the approach. They have also illuminated critical factors and conditions for particular consideration, most notably power.

Key theorists

We consider it important to trace six of the key theorists and concepts that contribute to the central thesis of critical pedagogy. This is by no means a comprehensive or exhaustive account. Further, these theorists cannot be separated from their historical settings, and this in itself demonstrates a key aspect of critical pedagogy – that all knowledge is socially and historically situated.

Whilst key theorists lived from 1920 to the current day in diverse situations, there are common threads throughout their ideas. They are all committed to democracy and social justice, and all believe that this can be achieved by increasing the awareness of all people of the use of power around them. For some the study is academic, for others the challenge needs to picked up by practitioners, and yet others focus on community settings for this valuable work.

Paulo Freire

Arguably, the most well-known and influential theorist was the South American educationalist Paulo Freire. Born in Brazil in the 1920s, at a time of a republic that featured oppression and marginalisation of masses of poor people, Freire realised that the masses living in Barrios were unable to participate in political processes such as voting because they could not access education and were illiterate. As a result Freire developed a literacy project where he ostensibly taught adult literacy, but was in reality doing so much more. The reading material used to develop literacy was real documents and information and as such was a meaningful activity focused around the adults' lives. Freire encouraged people to question what they had read, rather than accepting it at face value. They then began to question broader issues in their lives, such as why they were poor and why they had been denied access to education. The act of adult literacy was therefore deeply politicising and led to Freire having to leave the country to avoid imprisonment.

This form of education is the most tangible pre-cursor to critical pedagogy as we know it today and it was born out of acute oppression. The literacy project evoked the emancipation of the adults in that it helped them to read, which gave them greater understanding of what was going on around them. It gave them the education that the ruling classes had and thus access to more equitable rights to society. Equality is thus a key aspect of critical pedagogy, in the pursuit of social justice and wellbeing.

Critical pedagogy is a practice that the oppressed helped to develop; *with* not *for* the oppressed: "while no one liberates himself [sic] by his own efforts alone, nor is he [sic] liberated by others" (Freire, 1970: 35).

Freire's work hasn't been without critique. Of particular importance is the critique from feminism. As can be seen in the extracts taken from Freire's work, there is a clear dominant male perspective. For example, "the more accurately men [sic] grasp true causality...". Freire's initial works were written before second wave feminism. However, his later works addressed this and the benefits of feminist thought.

This did not stop many feminists being greatly influenced by Freire's works. Feminist educators have often cited Freire as the educational theorist who has come closest to the approach and goals of feminist pedagogy (Culley and Portuges, 1985). Weiler (1991) highlighted a shared vision of social transformation and argued that underlying both pedagogies were certain common assumptions concerning oppression, consciousness and historical change.

Henry Giroux

Giroux grew up in the United States some 20 years after Freire. Giroux became highly dissatisfied with the dominant forms of education in the US that served to control rather than liberate students. As such he has become a leading progressive educationalist and remains a prolific social commentator and author.

For Giroux, critical pedagogy is the key to overcoming such repression, enabling education to "mobilize students to be critically engaged agents, attentive to important social issues and alert to the responsibility of deepening and expanding the meaning and practices of a vibrant democracy" (Giroux, 2015: 14). Giroux, like Freire, demands that critical pedagogy leads to substantive action beyond awareness as it is only action that will lead to change.

Whilst Freire was provoked by the republic in Brazil, Giroux was confronted by Neoliberalism. This, he states, created economic Darwinism where the dispossessed and 'social dead' are consigned to frontier zones or put out of sight under the dominant principles of hyper-individualism, self-interest and consumerism (Giroux, 2011: 92). For Giroux, critical pedagogy is the key to change, as it leads people to awareness and action, and because politics starts when power is made visible (ibid: 134).

Giroux's perspective is important in justifying a critical approach to CYPF wellbeing, as it not only focuses in on education, but it draws out the key elements of awareness, choice and action, that our own research underpinning this book has found as the key process of empowerment and agency.

Philosopher John Searle (1990) criticises Giroux's goal as creating political radicals. This questions the antagonistic moral and political grounds of the ideals of critical pedagogy. It illuminates an inherent tension between varying moral perspectives and is also found in John Dewey's work in progressive education (although beyond the space and scope within this chapter).

Michel Foucault

Foucault was born in France in 1926 and was educated during the heyday of French existential philosophy, with Hegel and Marx as contemporary intellectuals. Foucault, like his contemporaries hated the bourgeois society and empathised with those who were marginalised. He became an academic in a range of French universities in the 1960s and became politically active in the 1970s, protesting on behalf of marginalised groups.

Although already alluded to within the arguments of the two previous theorists, Foucault provides an important perspective in the presentation of critical pedagogy, in his interest in forms and mechanisms of **power**. He analysed power in very specific contexts, such as mental health, sexuality and crime and punishment. From these studies he was able to develop three major ideas about power:

1   that of truth and the notion that there are several versions of the truth;
2   that of control and the notion that people control a preferred version of truth to dominate society; leading to
3   legitimisation and how people use their superiority to legitimise their truth.

Linking with the previous two theorists, we need to understand that there are multiple truths about an experience. What is important in critical pedagogy is to help CYPF understand their truth. Foucault's profound challenges to the nature of truth and the ways the powerful legitimise their version of the truth is deeply embedded in critical pedagogy, which argues all forms of truth as subjective and political.

Foucault has been criticised for rejecting the liberal values and philosophy associated with the Enlightenment, while simultaneously secretly relying on them (Biblio, 2016). Foucault took issue with this criticism noting that he believed strongly in human freedom and that his philosophy was a fundamentally optimistic one, as he believed that something positive could always be done no matter how bleak the situation.

Some historians have also criticised Foucault for his use of historical information, claiming that he frequently misrepresented things, got his facts wrong, or simply made them up entirely. Jacques Derrida wrote one of the most extensive critiques of Foucault's reading of Rene Descartes (Derrida, 1998: 60).

Antonio Gramsci

Working further with the notion of power, Gramsci was imprisoned for eleven years of his life by Mussolini because of his communist beliefs. In prison he developed an influential theory of power. Gramsci (1971) thought that capitalism had developed a 'manufactured consent', an invisible agreement in society about 'the ways things are around here'. This unconscious agreement about 'the way things are' was what he called 'hegemony'. This hegemony was often created and perpetuated by the bourgeois, or upper classes, legitimising the world as they saw it. This led to the idea of 'counter-hegemonic' struggles, where alternatives to dominant views of what is normal and legitimate are advanced.

Gramsci's work leads us to question the assumptions or taken for granted notions of 'the truth'. For example, it leads us to question the assumptions that particular forms of education are needed, that the pedagogy is appropriate and the extent to which it conforms to some invisible notion of the truth (such as racism and sexism). Efforts to identify and question dominant hegemonies remain a key part of critical pedagogy today.

In justifying a critical approach to working with CYPF wellbeing, it is important that we facilitate their identification and questioning of dominant hegemonies, rather than simply accept the status quo.

Saul Alinsky

Alinsky, born in 1909 in the United States, was an activist whose approach to activism was characterised by making people 'angry' enough to take action themselves. His key idea was community organising – a process by which people are brought together to act in common self-interest (Alinsky, 1946). He instigated a host of important and influential community groups such as the Industrial Areas Foundation. This was based on his core belief in humanity: "My only fixed truth is a belief in people, a conviction that if people have the opportunity to act freely and the power to control their own destinies, they'll generally reach the right decisions" (Alinksy, 1971).

Alinsky's antagonistic approach, which although important to learn from, is seen as incongruent with many people's approach. His core approach to activism of making people 'angry' enough to take action themselves (TIME, 1970) is the point at which many other people's arguments diverge. Awareness and critical consciousness are not necessarily always seen to equate to anger.

Maxine Greene

Greene, born in 1917 in the United States, was an internationally recognised educator and philosopher. Her reflective theories and social critiques have contributed to the democratic tradition of critical pedagogy. Her focus draws in the concepts of structure and agency, which are central in our argument here of wellbeing, structures being the enabling or constraining forces that surround us and agency being the extent to which people have awareness, make choices and act on those choices, in relation to the structures. Greene argues that if situations cannot be created that enable people to deal with feelings of being manipulated by outside forces, there will be far too little sense of agency among them. Further she argues that without a sense of agency, people are unlikely to pose significant questions, the existentially rooted questions, in which learning begins (Greene, 1988).

The Maxine Greene centre for Aesthetic Education and Social Imagination remains as a testament to her work. As the centre says, Maxine "explores living in awareness and 'wide-awakeness' in order to advance social justice" (2016). Greene uses the creative arts and literature to enable people to speak with their own voices (2009a) and to provoke social imagining with its questioning of, "what next" and "what can be done" (2009b). Her focus on awareness through dialogue and creativity and giving voice to those silenced had a major impact on critical pedagogy.

There are, of course, many critical pedagogues whose voices we have not been able to represent here and many have not received the publicity that they should in the wider world, most notably, bell hooks, Ira Shor and Joe Kinchloe. Two key factors led to the emergence of critical theory. These were John Dewey's principles of democratic education and the role of reflection in learning, the works of institutions such as The Frankfurt School's analysis of inequalities. A good account of these important voices can be found in Duncan-Andrade and Morrell (2008), suggested in further reading. The key principles from these theorists are summarised in the Table 4.1 below.

Reflective activity

Which of these key theorists have you heard of and align with?
Which do you challenge or disagree with?
What are the key concepts that particularly support your approach to practice?

Four key concepts of critical pedagogy

From the above we can draw out some key critical concepts that are central within critical pedagogy: oppression, power, critical consciousness and problematisation. These are each discussed in turn below.

Oppression

Oppression is a situation in which people are governed or treated in an unfair and cruel way and prevented from having opportunities and freedom. It is also the presumption in favour of dominant social groups that skews all social relationships and is encoded in their very structure (Sisneros *et al.*, 2008).

Key theorists have tackled this at a global level and challenged governance and the State in creating cultures of silence, which keep the dispossessed

Table 4.1 Key theorists and their principles of critical pedagogy

Key theorists	Principles adopted into critical pedagogy
Paulo Freire	Education that liberates Critical consciousness Problematising Dialogue Focus on human experiences
Michel Foucault	Games of truth Power is relational – one dominates, one submits 'Truth' is legitimised through supervision, control and correction
Antonio Gramsci	Hegemony
Maxine Greene	Giving people voice Reflection and learning through the arts Social imagining – what can be done, what next?
The Frankfurt School Scholars	Identification of power with critical theory
Ira Shor	Identified the repression and social control in schools in America

Henry Giroux	Identified the repression and social control in schools in
	   America
	Need for awareness and action in order to counter
	   neolibearlism

Joe Kinchloe	Established a global movement for critical pedagogy through Freire centres Sought to remove repression and social control from schools
John Dewey	Democratic education Reflection in learning

Margaret Ledwith	Identified the potential of critical pedagogy in community
	   settings
	Focused on developing collective action in community
	   settings

ignorant and lethargic. Freire, for example, suggests this ensures the position of victims of false generosity and paternalism, who learn to fear freedom and internalise their own oppression and are thus complicit in it. Yet a person's calling is to create liberty (Freire, 1970: 32).

This manifests for us as practitioners within the CYPF we work with on a daily basis, who are oppressed by people in their lives, living within particular historical social and cultural norms, enshrined within oppressive societal conditions. This is the fourth generation workless alcoholic young man on a court order; the young woman in care being groomed for sexual exploitation; the young carer doing their best to engage with their education in a seemingly rigid system; or the family on the edge of care, who considers any service the enemy as they will split the family up.

Essentially, this approach is based on political liberation and freedom from oppression. Freire argued that education should foster freedom among learners by enabling them to reflect on their world and thereby change it. This method requires CYPF not to recreate the world they find themselves in, but to become aware of reality, decontextualising it from everyday situations, in order to question and challenge the status quo.

Power

Foucault introduced, in the first instance, the notion of games of **truth** (1973). Foucault proposed there are several versions of 'the truth' in any situation. These versions of the truth may not align with everyone's 'reality' of the experience. These different versions of the truth can lead to different forms of domination as power is exerted. Think for a moment about sexuality – there are notions of what is 'normal' and 'okay' and therefore not 'okay' in different societies. Individuals may or may not sit in accordance with these norms. Which of these accounts is 'the truth'? How does a society's view of 'normal' sexuality impact on people who do not conform to those norms? If we see truth as a game, then we are perhaps more open to thinking of different sets of rules governing the players on the board and the ways that they privilege the winners and disadvantage the losers.

Foucault's second idea is that **control** is needed to ensure that the preferred version of 'the truth' dominates society (1978). Foucault (1982) conceptualised power as a series of actions that can incite, induce, seduce, release or contrive, and that make certain behaviours more or less probable. In other words, for Foucault, power was relational, it existed in the relationships between people, in their ability to convince or control, and in their agreement to conform to various forms of 'the truth', or to disagree and enter a power struggle (1980). This is seen in the traditional notion of the role of the formal educator and Freire's 'banking' concept of the educator's version of knowledge and truth being deposited into the mind of the learner. The educator is the holder of the knowledge and the learner is the passive recipient. The educator holds all control of the content, delivery method and timing, whereas the learner has no control over what they want to learn, when or how. This is of particular significance when discussed in terms of social justice and wellbeing, as we learn about the world and our place in it. Traditional education tells people their place; whereas critical pedagogy helps people discover their place.

This led to Foucault's third discovery of the number of ways people try to **legitimate** their 'truth' and their superiority over others through supervision, control and correction (Foucault, 1973: 70). In traditional education, there is only one truth; that of the teacher. This is legitimised through the power associated to their title, social conditions, rules and examination. We see this in the rhetoric of young people failing at school, rather than school failing young people.

This perspective is not only crucial in justifying a critical pedagogy to support CYPF wellbeing, but very challenging to some professionals. It challenges us to notice, reflect and question our awareness and use of power and that this is essential as it is inherently within all of us.

Critical consciousness

Freire's foundational claim was that intense reflection of oneself in relation to society, or conscientisation, was a necessary precursor to learning, growth, development, emancipation, and ultimately engaging in social change (Summerson Carr, 2016). Conscientisation has also been referred to as consciousness raising, or raising critical consciousness. Freire's approach uses the knowledge already possessed by people to give them the power to re-appropriate dominant knowledge for their own emancipation (Apple *et al.*, 2001). This can be seen as a growth in self-awareness, leading to questioning what may have previously been thought of as the norm, or how life had to be. This new knowledge of the world can lead to taking control of life towards one's own emancipation. Dirkx (1998) referred to this as a process in which learners developed the ability to analyse, pose questions and take action on the social, political, cultural and economic contexts that influenced and shaped their lives.

Freire's assumptions were that it was "associated directly to the transitivity of their consciousness" (1973: 37). He stated that "the more accurately men [sic] grasp true causality, the more critical their understanding of reality will be" (ibid: 39). He defined three levels of consciousness.

Magical consciousness is passive, unquestioning and adapts to reality:

> understanding will be magical to the degree that they fail to grasp causality ... simply apprehends facts and attributes to them a superior power by which it is controlled and to which it must therefore submit ... characterised by fatalism, which leads men [sic] to fold their arms, resigned to the impossibility of resisting the power of facts (ibid: 39).

CYPF may become resigned to the fact they have no control over their lives and no sense of other possibilities.

Naïve consciousness superimposes itself on reality:

> Naïve consciousness sees causality as a static, established fact, and thus is deceived in its perception (ibid: 39).

We have seen this within projects that aim to support young women at risk of sexual exploitation. Some young women are flattered by older men's attention and may seek to gain more of this through the way the men dictate, usually through sexualised behaviour. Some see men's attention to be their only way to find happiness and see their sexuality as their only asset. Some may see themselves as having agency, as they are choosing to use their sexuality to get the attention they want. However, this is based on a reality created by the men and that the only way to get their attention is through sexuality.

Critical consciousness is integrated with reality. This is a consciousness that has the power to transform reality because it identifies life's contradictions. If we continue with the above sexual exploitation example, we would see this in young women when they come to new understanding about the reality of the situation, usually in realising the older man is not in love with them, has other 'girlfriends', and that they are all being exploited. This may result in understanding other qualities in themselves and other realities in the world.

Freire (1972) defined pedagogy as substantively political; as educators we are also political agents. Education helps people to understand the world and prepares them to transform it, but only if we connect our work to the realities in which CYPF live (ibid). In critiquing the 'banking' concept of education, Freire educated towards critical consciousness so people became empowered to seek out understanding of how to make their lives better and therefore the lives of their community. This has profound implications for us as educators, trainers, facilitators, health care workers or youth workers, and more.

In our changing roles in differing partnerships and contexts, we need to understand, legitimise and promote our role in this process. A role that does not tell CYPF how to learn, grow or change; but listen and understand their lives so as to facilitate experiences where their knowledge about themselves and their lives could grow.

Problematisation

Critical pedagogy is in direct opposition to traditional, formal, 'banking' approaches to learning and development. Freire's work encourages us to think of our practice with CYPF as inherently political. It encourages the personal to become political, through engaging, questioning and challenging their world. This is through a process of 'problematisation' – building on the history and knowledge of CYPF and is the co-construction of knowledge through social interactions. This values and builds on previous experiences and shapes future ones. It places CYPF as experts of their own experience and thus knowledge. It personalises and contextualises learning and as such is experiential, again drawing parallels with the works of John Dewey.

Through dialogue (both between the learner and the facilitator and between the learner and their knowledge), it involves asking why the world is as it is and therefore problematises knowledge (Freire, 1972). Our role is therefore not 'teacher', but a 'teacher-learner', as we learn with the CYPF about their experience and knowledge. We are listeners, questioners, problem solvers, and a resource for CYPF to draw from. Likewise CYPF are not solely learners, but also teachers as they contribute their learning to the discussion (Freire, 1972). They too, listen, share, question, problem solve and seek out our resource to help.

This draws further from Alinsky's work that valued the non-expert listening approach. He states that the first thing community workers should do is listen, not talk, and learn to eat, sleep, breathe only one thing: the problems and aspirations of the community. He suggests that no matter how imaginative your tactics, how shrewd your strategy, you're doomed before you even start if you don't win the trust and respect of the people. The only way to get that is for you to trust and respect them, learning about them through immersion with them. Without that respect, Alinsky states, there's no communication, no mutual confidence and no action (Alinksy, 1971).

The distinction between a teacher and a learner is a clear example of a dichotomy. Freire, drawing on Marx's (1853) theory of consciousness, deliberately tried to see such terms in relation to one another rather than in contrast to one another. This is called dialectical theory. Teacher and learner are therefore brought together in relationship. Therefore, theory and practice are also brought together under the term praxis. Freire strived to ensure that theory was built from people's lived experiences (practice) and likewise that theory informed how people were able to live their lives. The two exist and inform one another rather than remaining distinct. The idea of praxis is central to critical pedagogy.

Souto-Manning (2010: 9) adds, "By problematizing, contesting language and concepts within specific contexts and taking socio-historical and cultural issues into account, one gains power to appropriate language, and utilise it to promote change". This problematising and dialogical process are key in critical pedagogy.

Freire proposes that this style of learning is liberating as opposed to traditional notions of learning that deposited knowledge or tell people how it should be. Critical pedagogy, in contrast, is a liberating form of working with CYPF.

The key aspects of these theories are summarised in Table 4.2 below to give more shape to critical pedagogy.

Critical pedagogy is based on the use of personal experiences as the learning resources, the problematisation of power, the consciousness raising supports CYPF to become critical citizens, self-determining and agentic. When this kind of work happens in groups, the personal experiences are often validated by others, shared with others, and the personal therefore becomes both political and collective.

Margaret Ledwith focuses on the transformative potential of critical pedagogy in community settings. Ledwith (2005) states that: "People make critical connections when they link culture, political, social and economic issues with their everyday life experience. This counters the apathy and passivity symptomatic of a culture of silence" (2005: 59). This perspective speaks to recent UK rhetoric of the Big Society. The principles of this are described below.

Table 4.2 Summary of key concepts of critical pedagogy

Theory	Principles defining critical pedagogy
Cultural politics	Teachers (in the broadest sense) must consider what they teach, how it is taught and how it reproduces power.
Socio-historical knowledge	All knowledge is created in specific social, cultural and historical settings. What is known, and who knows it therefore needs to be considered within that setting rather than seen as neutral.
Socially constructed knowledge	Knowledge is created by people in specific social, cultural and historical settings. People's individual stories therefore need to be understood in order to know what they know.
Dialectical theory	Knowledge is not a set of competing binaries, but is dialectical. Apparently opposing factors are in relationship with one another in a tension with contradictions that can only be understood by problematising rather than simplifying knowledge.
Praxis	The theory and practice divide is a prominent dichotomy that critical pedagogy rejects. Rather it embraces the two as mutually important, mutually reinforcing dialectic. Reflection is a key process to bringing theory into practice, and practice into theory.
Ideological critique	People's knowledge and beliefs is often presented as 'the truth', this is called ideology. Critical pedagogy seeks to reveal what different ideologies are at play in any situation.
Hegemony	Ideology is kept in place through social control applied by the dominant called hegemony. Critical pedagogy is committed to revealing hegemony at play. Counter-hegemony refers to efforts by the oppressed to overcome the ideology they are subjected to. Critical pedagogy is innately counter-hegemonic.

Vignette 4.1 The Big Society

In 2010 the UK Coalition Government stated their intention to build a 'Big Society'. They aimed to put more power and opportunity into people's hands, de-centralising government and empowering people to have more control of their destinies (Cabinet Office, 2010). The Government stated they want to give citizens, communities and local government the power and information they need to come together, solve the problems they face and build the Britain they want. They emphasised the desire for society, the families, networks, neighbourhoods and communities that form the fabric of so much of our everyday lives, to be bigger and stronger than ever before. Advocating that only when people and communities are given more power and take more responsibility can we achieve fairness and opportunity for all.

Opportunities of the Big Society

Coote (2010) highlighted that the principles of the Big Society were that people have assets, not just problems. This combined with a belief that when people are given the chance and treated as if they are capable, they tend to find they know what is best for themselves and can fix their own problems and hence efforts to get more people working together to run their own affairs locally. Coote goes on to outline the opportunities inherent within the successful implementation of these principles, such as better outcomes through co-production (people working together with shared power, e.g. increasing pupils' involvement in behaviour management processes); increased wellbeing, at both personal and collective levels; and increased social capital. The opportunities identified by Coote parallel the argument put forward in this chapter. This theoretical potential was important to remember amid the mass critique that ensued.

Critique of the Big Society

Coote (2010) encouraged engagement in critical debate and attempted to unpack what the Big Society actually was. However, there was initially little critique of the agenda (de St Croix, 2011), perhaps because it came about so quickly, or perhaps because of confusion over exactly what it meant.

Taking a critical stance to unpack this reveals that what the Big Society represents is far from the Freirean perspective presented within this chapter.

Ledwith (2011) drew further from Coote's work, suggesting that when people have control over what is happening in their lives, their health and wellbeing improves. However, she was critical of the policy that led to dismantling the established network of supporting voluntary and community sector organisations by withdrawing funding. Arguably the 'small state' and Big Society approach could appear congruent with social justice at face value, but it was also a challenging approach that could not be achieved through cuts; it needed to be invested in.

Ledwith (2011: 25) argued that "the small state is absolving its democratic responsibilities to the poorest in society by making austerity cuts in public services at the same time as making the poorest responsible for their own poverty". She further points out that the agenda is strong on the rhetoric of empowerment and weak on equality, continuing, "the poorest communities with the least resources will be faced with the biggest responsibilities" (p. 1). They have the biggest responsibilities because they have the most problems and the highest disadvantage. The Government could be viewed as abandoning the most disadvantaged with the cuts, taking away a skilled workforce and the agents of social change needed to develop 'dynamic' social capital and mobility.

This highlights concerns of how social capital will grow in these circumstances; how will CYPF find their way out of oppression, poverty and crime;

how will they live up to all that the Government expect them to live up to and contribute to the Big Society? The Government cuts removed the potential of their contribution and their freedom from oppression. Critical pedagogy is crucial in this process, yet is missing from the Big Society agenda.

The Big Society did little to address the structures that create poverty; in fact it was seen to add to the ever-widening social divisions. The banking crisis and world recession that created these cuts appeared to be being paid for by those most disadvantaged. Ledwith (2011) suggests that this will lead to those communities most marginalised, disadvantaged and dis-empowered not being able to survive, whereas those most privileged, powerful and advantaged will flourish.

Further critique, such as Norman (2010), has suggested that the Big Society is a cover up on a severe reduction in national and local state-provided services, masked by a cheery demand that volunteers step forward to provide them for free. The implications of voluntary work are a worrying prospect, as specialist areas of work, such as this book explores, are devalued and de-professionalised.

As practitioners we need to be critically aware of the policy surrounding our practice. We should not simply accept policy, because it is the only "new idea" (de St Croix, 2011: 44). We should make sure we are critical in order to truly understand our practice. If working from a critical pedagogy perspective, practitioners themselves need critical consciousness in order to facilitate CYPF critical consciousness. The 'feel good' factor elicited by the Big Society rhetoric is an example of how easily we can be drawn into mandated policy models.

Critical pedagogy is crucial in developing social justice and enhanced wellbeing, yet, as this vignette exemplifies, has been missing from policy. In not accepting the Big Society agenda at face value and critically questioning it, it illuminated the potential that the agenda was actually a contradiction. Power was de-centralised, as the Government stated, but responsibility landed with the most disempowered, with the least resource to make change. Critical pedagogy was diluted and distorted and not valued in the Big Society agenda.

Summary of key points

This chapter has outlined an approach to wellbeing defined by the social justice lens through which we are looking at it. Critical pedagogy is grounded in a social and educational vision of justice, equality and the belief that our work to support CYPF to learn, grow and develop is inherently political. Key theorists have developed critical concepts that underpin a critical approach. Firstly, these theorists' works were all founded based on the assumption of oppression being present. This is significant to our discussion of wellbeing and social justice, as it is concerned with how people have agency to negotiate potentially oppressive structures that cause, or are caused by, social injustice. This is considered more critically in the second key concept of power, in which the different ways in which oppression can manifest is critically explored. Therefore, the third central concept of critical pedagogy is its focus upon critical consciousness, where people become aware of oppression and power, realise there is choice in this and act on this in having agency within these structures, as well as finding enabling structures. Lastly, problematisation is seen as a key concept, or method, of achieving critical consciousness.

Reflective activity

How have you experienced key policies in practice?
Are you able to work from a critical approach, amid key agendas or budgetary cut backs?
Are you able to bring this approach to working with new partners and how is this received?

Further reading

Boal, A. *Theatre of the Oppressed.* New York: Routledge.
Darder, A., Baltodano, M., and Torres, R. (2009), *The Critical Pedagogy Reader*, 2nd edn. New York: Routledge.
Duncan-Andrade, J., and Morrell, E. (2008). *Possibilities for Moving from Theory to Practice in Urban Schools.* New York: Peter Lang Publishing.
Mullender, A., Ward, D., and Fleming, J. (2013). *Empowerment in Action. Self-directed Groupwork.* Basingstoke: Palgrave Macmillan.

References

Alinksy, S. D. (1946). *Reveille for Radicals.* Chicago: University of Chicago Press.
Alinksy, S. D. (1971). *Rules for Radicals.* New York: Random House.
Apple, M. W., Gandin, L. A., and Hypolito, A. M. (2001). 'Paulo Freire, 1921–97', in Bresler, L., Cooper, D., Palmer, J. (eds) *Fifty Modern Thinkers on Education – From Piaget to the Present.* London: Routledge, pp. 128–132.
Biblio (2016). 'Michel Foucault'. Accessed on 24. 9. 16 at http://biblio.co.uk/michel-foucault/author/226
Cabinet Office (2010). *Building the Big Society.* London: Cabinet Office.
Coote, A. (2010). *Ten Big Questions about the Big Society and Ten Ways to Make the Best of It.* London: nef.
Culley, M., and Portuges, C. (eds) (1985). *Gendered Subjects: the Dynamics of Feminist Teaching.* Boston: Routledge and Kegan Paul.
Derrida, J. (1998). *Resistances of Psychoanalysis*, translated by P. Kamuf, P. A. Brault and M. Naas. Stanford: Stanford University Press.
Dewey, J. (1963) *Experience and Education.* New York: Collier.

Dirkx, J. M. (1998). 'Transformative Learning Theory in the Practice of Adult Education: An Overview', *PAACE Journal of Lifelong Learning*, 7, 1–14.

Foucault, M. (1973). 'Truth and Juridical Forms', lecture in the University of Rio de Janeiro. Translated by R. Hurley, in Faubion, J. (ed) *'Power' Essential Works of Foucault 1954–1984 Volume 3*. London: Penguin, pp. 1–89.

Foucault, M. (1978). 'Governmentality', translated by R. Hurley, in Faubion, J. (ed.) *'Power' Essential Works of Foucault 1954–1984 Volume 3*. London: Penguin, pp. 201–222.

Foucault, M. (1980). *Power and Knowledge*. Translated by C. Gordon. Hemel Hempstead: Harvester Wheatsheaf.

Foucault, M. (1982). 'The Subject and Power', translated by R. Hurley, in Faubion, J. (ed.) *'Power' Essential Works of Foucault 1954–1984 Volume 3*. London: Penguin, pp. 326–348.

Freire, P. (1970). *The Pedagogy of the Oppressed*. New York: Seabury.

Freire, P. (1972). *Cultural Action for Freedom*. London: Penguin.

Freire, P. (1973). *Education as the Practice of Freedom in Education for Critical Consciousness*. New York: Continuum.

Freire, P. (1974). *Education for Critical Consciousness*. London: Continuum.

Giroux, H. (2011). *On Critical Pedagogy*. New York: Bloomsbury.

Giroux, H. (2015). 'Beyond Pedagogies of Represssion', *Monthly Review*, 67(10), 1.

Gramsci, A. (1971). *Selections from the Prison Notebooks of Antonio Gramsci*. New York: International Publishers.

Greene, M. (1988). *The Dialectics of Freedom*. New York: Teachers College Press.

Greene, M. (2009a). 'In Search of a Critical Pedagogy', in Darder, A., Baltodano, M., and Torres, R. (eds), *The Critical Pedagogy Reader*, 2nd edn. New York: Routledge, pp. 97–114.

Greene, M. (2009b) 'The Arts and the Search for Social Justice'. Accessed on 24. 9. 16 at https://maxinegreene.org/uploads/library/arts_n_search_4_social_justice.pdf

Kinchloe, J. (2005). *Critical Pedagogy*. New York: Peter Lang.

Ledwith, M. (2005). *Community Development: A Critical Approach*. London: Polity Press.

Ledwith, M. (2011). *Community Development: A Critical Approach*, 2nd edn. London: Polity Press.

Maxine Greene Center for Aesthetic Education and Social Imagination (2016). 'About Maxine Green'. Accessed on 24. 9. 16 at: https://maxinegreene.org/about/maxine-greene

Norman, J. (2010). 'The Big Society', *The Independent*, 21. 11. 2010. Accessed on 22. 4. 17 at: http://www.independent.co.uk/arts-entertainment/books/reviews/the-big-society-by-jesse-norman-2136907.html

de St Croix, T. (2011). 'Struggles and Silences: Policy, Youth Work and the National Citizen Service', *Youth and Policy*, 106, 43–59.

Searle, J. (1990). 'The Storm Over the University', *The New York Review of Books*, December 6, 1990.

Sisneros, J., Stakeman, C., Joyner, M. C., and Schmitz, C. L. (2008). *Critical Multicultural Social Work*. Chicago: Lyceum Books, Inc.

Souto-Manning, M. (2010). *Freire, Teaching and Learning. Culture Circles Across Contexts*. New York: Peter Lang.

Summerson-Carr, E. (2016). 'Rethinking Empowerment Theory Using a Feminist Lens: The Importance of Process', *Affilia*, 18(1), 8–20.

TIME (1970). 'Essay: Radical Saul Alinksy: Prophet of Power to the People', *Time Magazine*, March 2, 1970. Accessed 27. 6. 16 at http://content.time.com/time/maga zine/article/0,9171,904228,00.html

Weiler, K. (1991). 'Freire and a Feminist Pedagogy of Difference', *Harvard Educational Review*, 61(4), 449–474.

5 Wellbeing, structures and post-structuralism

Chapter overview

Structuralism is the view that people are created, shaped and ruled by the environments and societies in which they live; they are structured by them (Durkheim, 1982). This chapter provides examples of this form of thinking and the theorists who led this line of sociology are described. Power is highlighted as the core feature of all structures and its key features explored.

Structuralism

Structuralist views emerged from the age of scientific thought in the 18th and 19th centuries. Jeffery (2011: 8) suggests that society was seen as separate and distinct from individuals: "Society was seen as a force outside the individual which curbed, restrained and shaped their actions". People were seen to be subjected to societal rules, highlighted by Rousseau (1762: 3) who said, "Man is born free, but everywhere is in chains".

Structuralism states that structures are dominant forces acting on people. Structuralism also positions people in a very particular way; as objects sharing identical qualities. Jeffery (ibid.) adds that in essence, individuals had no real individuality, but were "reducible to various common shared characteristics". This era of thought is best characterised as seeing humans as automatons, or robots, that did what was willed of them by society.

Durkheim was one of the key proponents of structuralism. He stated that people are controlled and created by society – they merely occupy roles (Durkheim, 1982). From this functionalist stance institutions, groups and individuals all had functions to fulfil that sustained and upheld the state and society. Anyone who stepped out of their role was seen as deviant and a threat to society. This can be seen as objectivist, as people are seen as 'objects' rather than 'subjects' of their own lives. From this perspective they can be manipulated in the interests of society whose needs are always construed, according to Durkheim, to be paramount. Durkheim's views were perhaps extreme, over-emphasising the role of the state over individuals. This perspective was also unable to account for how structures were established in the first place, and how they could be changed or mediated over time.

Parsons (1937) developed Durkheim's work. He maintained that 'structures' dominated, but granted people capacity to be 'actors' choosing to maintain or change the social order as a voluntary activity. He suggested that people decided to 'volunteer' to fulfil these roles or not and created his principal of voluntarism (1937: 369). By accepting prescribed roles and norms, people would maintain the status quo. Whilst people are bestowed with some choice here, and Parsons acknowledged people's psychological factors, it is a limited choice as to which prescribed role in society to fulfil, with societal issues also positioned as prevailing. This theory was again criticised, as it could not account for societal change. It was also inherently classist, as Parsons saw the elite dominant classes as upholding society as the lower classes were not viewed intelligent enough to understand the situation (Parsons, 1937: 279–281).

Max Weber's (1978) account of society bestowed individuals with a more active role within structures. He too stressed that individuals existed and acted within social contexts that were of prime importance. However, he proposed people had a role in choosing how to act and in constructing society. This acknowledged that people did interact in structures. To some extent, Weber was a bridge between the structuralist movement and that of agency – featured in the next chapter.

Structures and systems

So what exactly are structures? They are all the factors that control what we do – for good and for bad. These include norms, rules, laws, discourses and cultures. **Norms** are the things that are taken for granted – your family will have norms around when to wash the pots after eating. If someone comes in and breaks that **rule** then it is noticed. **Laws** are straightforward – but it is probably worth noting that there can be informal laws and rules and legal ones. The term **discourses** means the language and imagery that is used in reference to something. For young people, for example, there was a clear discourse that prevailed in the UK of anti-social young people wearing hoodies, hanging out in gangs, yobs, thugs, and such, terrorising society. Young people like this did perhaps exist, but the prevalence of this 'discourse' meant that this was how every young person was thought of. Equally, families needing any form of benefit have been collectively thought of as lazy, work-shy, welfare scroungers and the image of a few is used to describe all. **Culture** refers to the collection of norms and rules that create 'the way that things are done around here'. A clear example of this within children's services is the new neoliberal culture of paperwork and bureaucracy. Paperwork and form filling are now criticised and thought of as being prevalent 'everywhere'.

This in turn, links to the concept of **systems**. Jeffery (2011: 6) states that systems are recurring elements of society that act to sustain it. This combines the "practices that underpin the effective functioning of our society, with structures referring to the properties of these systems". An aversion to risk within society and a culture of fear (Furedi, 2007) creates a system that accepts and perpetuates the above example of paperwork, that evidences every effort has been made to keep CYPF safe.

These structures are invisible; they are a tacit part of our world. Although they are largely invisible, they are not magical. They are a direct result of actions to create structures that propose to ensure the smooth running of society.

All of these different structures and discourses exist at multiple levels; in friendships, families, communities, areas, countries and globally. These are shown in Figure 5.1 below.

This nested presentation relates well to Bronfenbrenner's (1994) bio-ecological model of child development. This model accounted for all the different environmental factors in which a person or child interacts. The account suggested the need to take account of the influences of environmental factors on human development. This model obviously resonates with the description of structures in this chapter, and can be seen as a tool with which we might map structures, so that we can then decide how to work with them, rather than unconsciously being subjugated to them.

Structuralists believe that structures, at all of these different levels, act on people shaping what they do. The structures can either act on people in a positive way – **enabling** them to do what they want, or they can act on them in a negative way, **constraining** them. The discourses are also not always aligned, so we can experience conflicting discourses. The table below illustrates some common discourses about young people that can directly contrast with one another.

Reflective activity

Have you ever experienced any of these conflicting discourses?
What tensions has each one created for you?
Who dictates these different perspectives?
How do you reconcile them?
What others exist?

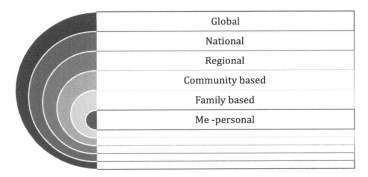

Figure 5.1 Nested layers of structures

Table 5.1 Conflicting youth discourses

Enabling discourses		Constraining discourses
Listen to young people	Versus	Centralised planning
Youth voice and experience	Versus	Objective evidence
Needs-led services	Versus	Predetermined outcomes
Young responsible citizens	Versus	Deficit youth and a culture of fearing young people
Adultification	Versus	Paternalism
Safeguarding	Versus	You're to blame

Sociology offers accounts of structures at three main levels – the macro, meso and micro. These are perhaps easier to think of than the six levels in Figure 5.1. **Macro**-sociology examines social structures (Durkheim, 1982; Marx, 1990; Parsons, 1951), whereas **micro**-sociology examined daily social interactions (Weber, 1947 and Garfinkel, 1967). **Meso**-level forces of social control sit between the two and consist of organisational and community-based influences (Turner, 2006).

For practitioners the micro-level structures might constitute individual and team enabling and constraining factors, for example, Social Workers or Key Workers with increasing and complex family case loads. At a meso, or middle level, structures are organisational, cultural norms and hierarchical structures. For example, new multi-agency working and enforced targets. Macro structures refer to the larger societal messages, and political context in which we operate, for example, the 'Troubled families' agenda and related policy.

A good example of discourses at work is provided in Blackmore's (1999) classic feminist analysis of educational leadership. Blackmore evidenced the power of the leadership discourse in the 1990s to create norms of performativity, strong leadership, entrepreneurialism, discipline, hierarchy, accountability, efficiency and line management. These constrained the availability of other, more feminine, forms of leadership. It seems as if this trend has continued into the current decade. Ledwith (2005) identifies these societal messages as 'hegemony', or the dominance of a few over the masses (hegemony is discussed further below). Such mechanisms of control can be maintained and modified, wittingly or unwittingly, by practitioners (ibid: 121).

Similarly, Wearing (1998: 61) defines hegemony as "the control of the consciousness by cultural dominance through the institutions of society". Wearing adds that "power and privilege are maintained through cultural hegemony, but struggles over hegemonic control are inevitable". When a discourse becomes hegemonic, it drops out of conscious awareness and becomes invisible. Deliberate thought is needed to reveal these hidden hegemonic discourses and this is, in part, the role of critical pedagogy.

Reflective activity

Think about a typical day.

What do you do? Make a list of all your daily tasks.

Now think about all the structures that might have had an influence on why you do that.

Even your choice of clothes and style of driving might be the result of particular discourses.

Have fun, and don't feel too spooked by the results – don't worry, you are not a robot!

Power

What is common in all of these structures, and inherent in structuralism, is power. All structures exert power on people. Therefore we must consider theories of power in this context. You will already be aware of some of the issues of power from having read chapter 4 on social justice and critical pedagogy. Here, we summarise some of the key aspects of power and how these relate to structures.

Sources of power

Gramsci (1971) thought that capitalist society had unconsciously 'manufactured consent' on how society would run. For example, buying and selling goods rather than exchanging them for free is an unspoken rule of capitalism. This invisible agreement about 'the ways things are around here' is called '**hegemony**'.

As introduced in chapter 4, Gramsci (1971) pointed out that hegemonic views were created and perpetuated by the bourgeois, or upper classes, legitimising the world as they saw it. This is clearly an issue for social justice. In response, the lower subjugated classes often engage in 'counter-hegemonic' struggles, where alternatives to dominant views of what is normal and legitimate are advanced.

The dominant hegemony is one layer of structure that will enable and constrain CYPF's wellbeing and social justice.

Technologies of power

Foucault (1973) was interested in how power worked, he wanted to establish its technologies and mechanisms. In order to reveal these, Foucault studied power in specific contexts; mental asylums, sexuality and crime and punishment. From these studies he was able to develop three major ideas about power.

As detailed in the previous chapter, the 'game of truth' is Foucault's (1973: 2–5) first technology of power. Foucault proposes that there are always several versions of 'the truth' in any situation which may not align with the 'reality' of experience. These different versions of the truth lead to different forms of domination as they exert power over people. For example, 'welfare scrounging' is one version of the truth in the welfare state in the UK, which oppresses all of those who receive benefits. If we see truth as a game, then we are perhaps more open to thinking of different sets of rules governing the players on the board, as well as the ways that these rules privilege the winners and disadvantage the losers.

The second technology of power is social control. This control is needed to ensure that dominant groups' preferred version of 'the truth' takes hold in society. In order to legitimise dominant views, surveillance, supervision and correction exist (1973: 70). In the modern day we are beset by arguments about the extent to which the state can monitor people's daily lives through CCTV footage, internet and phone records, and credit card transactions. These are state systems of surveillance and supervision and there will be other systems that exist in your workplaces to ensure that you work within agreed tacit and explicit boundaries.

Various versions of the truth compete with one another, and the power of people to establish their version as dominant lies in their actions. Foucault (1982: 341) documented the ways in which people incite, induce, seduce, contrive, fight or manipulate. These actions are examples of what Foucault sees as the relational nature of power. The game of truth and social control existed in an unconscious contest between people for superiority – power struggles.

Games of truth, surveillance, supervision and control and power struggles are another layer of structure that will enable or constrain wellbeing and social justice in any setting.

Powerful people

The rich or bourgeois used to be considered the powerful people in a country, but this has changed dramatically over time. Owen Jones (2015) provides a thorough account of the ways in which 'the establishment' in the UK controls others through the use of discourse. Powerful holders include: the state, the business elite, media and police, all of whom control what is considered 'the truth'. He draws attention to the language of 'tough decisions' used by politicians, which usually equates to a reduction in the living standards of others. Such 'tough decisions' are usually tough for anyone other than the politicians making them and powerfully imply that anyone who questions them is weak or cowardly (2015: 63). Jones's account of the ways in which structures of power are maintained reveals who invests in maintaining the current and deeply unjust societal status quo.

We are all enmeshed in a range of structures. State structures, from the establishment, are perhaps the most powerful and can enable and constrain wellbeing and social justice in profound ways. Is there no hope then? Are the oppressed powerless victims in the face of these types, technologies and protagonists? We think not. And our approach advocates, not!

Firstly, the people at the top are usually there because, at some point, the people below them have endorsed them to be there. Political parties are elected by people voting in the UK. This means that people have power. If people collectively voice their counter-hegemonic views, and make it clear that they will vote for politicians who represent those views then, theoretically, they can effect change. Secondly, as the world becomes more technologically connected there are new technologies of power emerging. Counter-hegemonic social media campaigns, petitions and demonstrations can be organised globally at the click of a button, increasing awareness more widely and challenging discourses. This is shifting power away from the people in higher hierarchical positions, to those with mass voice.

The following chapters on agency and empowerment will look further into how people reclaim this power to effect change.

Positioning of power

Jeffery (2011: 17) presents a lively account of the changes to social work in the UK and the way it has positioned service users. She describes how the helping professions initially "denied the reality of client responsibility, with social workers viewing their clients' behaviour as socially deviant, or the result of mental illness". The social worker's role was very much about helping the client to conform to societal norms – an oppressive process. A further critique of the helping professions was of **assistencialism**. This means that practitioners treated people as passive objects, able to receive help, but not able to help themselves – people needed to be assisted.

Another way in which dominant groups protect themselves is in positioning non-dominant individuals and groups as 'others' (Said, 1978). The process of 'othering' defines threatening groups by what is different. This binary way of thinking divides citizens into two groups – us and others, haves and have-nots, included and excluded, practitioners and service users. This objectification is unhelpful; it creates structures that can limit agency through the invalidation of identity and experience (Said, 1978). This process is often initiated by the media and politicians who seek to define an underclass who need support or who need keeping in their place and this becomes the space of policy intervention. The process of 'othering' can therefore be seen as an essential component of politics – without them there would be no need for policy and no need for politicians.

Thankfully a client-centred approach emerged in 1960s stressing the need for mutually respectful relationships between the client and the worker rather than the hierarchical ones that had previously existed. The client-centred approach stressed the role of the individual in being experts in their own lives with the capacity to change (Rogers, 1961; Kelly, 1955).

Two decades later, the radical social work movement emerged in the UK, alongside pressure groups that championed the rights of people. The radical movement went to the far left and positioned society as the villain that caused the difficulties experienced by clients (Bailey and Brake, 1975). The 'casework' approach that described clients and their need for 'treatment' was critiqued, as was social work itself, as a form of oppression (Jeffery, 2011: 20). More recently, the agenda of 'participation' and then 'co-production' challenge professional wisdom, and redistribute it to service users. This drive has seen services' design informed by service users as the experts in what matters.

Whilst these may be viewed as 'political positions', they are significant in the agency that they bestow service users with. Politically 'right' views tend to treat service users as deviants in need of treatment, whereas 'left' views treat them as victims of an oppressive society. Services themselves therefore become structures that enable or constrain the agency of service users by the nature of the position that they bestow on them.

Practitioners also operate within structures. For some these are experienced as oppressive, rotten and at fault. The rise of managerialism in the UK, for example, has led to increased practitioner time dedicated to paperwork rather than client work. This can lead to practitioners who are 'acting out their prescribed role as servants of the state' and 'feel powerless in their inability to change anything' (Jeffery, 2011: 35). This may particularly be the case for practitioners who view society as the site of all ills, working within a system that views service users as deviants. In this situation they may feel that their practice is a mere sticking plaster over the deep-seated social injustice of the world. This is known as placatory practice.

Vignette 5.1 The UK Troubled Families Policy

The Troubled Families agenda (Home Office, 2014) in the UK is a clear example of a policy both positioning people in a certain way and controlling what people do. The very name of the policy 'troubled families' implies that families are simultaneously or alternatively in trouble, experiencing trouble or causing trouble themselves. This is a negative and unhelpful positioning of 120,000 families in the UK. Secondly the policy defines a narrow set of behaviours that define a 'troubled family' and also, by default, the areas of work that must be engaged in to move them 'out of trouble'. These include: parents out of work, children out of school, high levels of crime and anti-social behaviour and resultant high costs to the state. The assumption is that these families are at fault. There is no acknowledgement that the structures of work may prevent them from being employed, the structures of schooling may prevent engagement and that the structures of society may predispose people to crime. Rather the structures are positioned as acceptable norms and the families that are not abiding by them as deviant.

The families are defined as so 'troubled' and 'troubling' that the Home Office publication is even titled – *'Tackling Troubled Families'*, creating an expectation of difficulty and adversity for any helping profession wanting to get involved. This is not the most positive start to any working relationship with a family.

Summary of key points

Structures exist explicitly and implicitly in every context and situation. These structures act on people. It is important to remember that structures both enable and constrain rather than only focusing on what they stop us from doing. The structures exist at many levels, locally, nationally and globally. Some structures may be the same globally; however, they tend to be culturally and temporally situated. They are complex and mutually reinforce or contradict one another. As a result we may find ourselves subordinated or privileged by a range of structures at once. No matter where they are located, the structures work through power. Power is created through relationships and repeated dominant discourses that become hegemonic. Systems of surveillance and supervision are used by the establishment to keep them all in place.

Mann (1985: 72) proposes that this emphasis on structure only tells half the story: "In order to explain how men and women make history in particular circumstances we need an account sensitive enough to detangle human agency from structural effect". It is to this task that the next chapter turns.

Further reading

Burr, V. (1995). *An Introduction to Social Constructionism*. London: Routledge.
Foucault, M. (1982). 'The Subject and Power'. Translated by R. Hurley, in Faubion, J. (ed.) *'Power' Essential Works of Foucault 1954–1984 Volume 3*. London: Penguin, pp. 326–348.
Furedi, F. (2007). *The Politics of Fear*. London: Bloomsbury Press.
Jones, O. (2015). *The Establishment and How They Get Away With It*. London: Sage.
Ledwith, M. (2016). *Community Development in Practice*. Bristol: Policy Press.

References

Bailey, R., and Brake, M. (eds) (1975). *Radical Social Work*. London: Edward Arnold.
Blackmore, J. (1999). *Troubling Women. Feminism, Leadership and Educational Change*. Buckingham: Open University Press.
Bronfenbrenner, U. (1994). 'Ecological Models of Human Development', *International Encyclopaedia of Education*, Vol. 3. 2nd edn. Oxford: Elsevier, pp. 1643–1647.
Durkheim, E. (1982). *The Rules of Sociological Method*. New York: Free Press.
Foucault, M. (1973). 'Truth and Juridical Forms', lecture in the University of Rio de Janeiro. Translated by R. Hurley, in Faubion, J. (ed.) *'Power' Essential Works of Foucault 1954–1984 Volume 3*. London: Penguin, pp. 1–89.
Foucault, M. (1982). 'The Subject and Power'. Translated by R. Hurley, in Faubion, J. (ed.) *'Power' Essential Works of Foucault 1954–1984 Volume 3*. London: Penguin, pp. 326–348.
Furedi, F. (2007). *The Politics of Fear*. London: Bloomsbury Press.
Garfinkel, H. (1967). *Studies in Ethnomethodology*. Englewood Cliffs, NJ: Prentice Hall.
Gramsci, A. (1971). *Selections from the Prison Notebooks of Antonio Gramsci*. New York: International Publishers.

Home Office (2014). *Tackling Troubled Families – Have You Got What it Takes?* London: Home Office.

Jeffery, L. (2011). *Understanding Agency.* Bristol: Policy Press.

Jones, O. (2015). *The Establishment and How They Get Away With It.* London: Sage.

Kelly, G. A. (1955). *The Psychology of Personal Constructs.* New York: Norton.

Ledwith, M. (2005). *Community Development: A Critical Approach.* London: Policy Press.

Mann, K. (1985). 'The Making of a Claiming Class: The Neglect of Agency in Analyses of the Welfare State', *Critical Social Policy,* 5(15), pp. 62–74.

Marx, K. (1990). *Capital. A Critique of Political Economy. Volume One* (trans. Ben Fowkes). London: Penguin Books.

Parsons, T. (1937). *The Structure of Social Action.* New York: McGraw Hill.

Parsons, T. (1951). *The Social System.* New York: The Free Press.

Rogers, C. (1961). *On Becoming a Person.* New York: Mariner Books.

Rousseau, E. (1762). *The Social Contract.* Amsterdam: Marc Michel Rey.

Said, E. (1978). *Orientalism.* New York: Random House.

Turner, B. (2006). *Vulnerability and Human Rights.* Pennsylvania, PA: Pennsylvania State University Press.

Wearing, B. (1998). *Leisure and Feminist Theory.* London: Sage.

Weber, M. (1947). *The Theory of Social and Economic Organisation.* Translated by T. Parsons and A. Morrell Henderson. New York: The Free Press.

Weber, M. (1978). *Economy and Society.* Berkeley, CA: University of California Press.

6   Wellbeing and agency

Chapter overview

This chapter introduces agency, defining it as CYPF ability to be aware of the world around them, to choose a course of action and to act on it, creating the world that they want. Building on the previous chapter's description of structures around us, this chapter shows theorists who privilege an agency perspective, presenting the view that people create societies. This is explored from psychological and sociological perspectives. The benefits and limitations of this agentic approach are identified. The chapter concludes by presenting a balanced view of structure and agency as a dualism rather than as a duality. Agency is the state that people need to possess in order to have wellbeing and in order to create a more socially just world.

What is agency?

Agency refers to the awareness, choices and actions of an individual. It is often referred to as 'human agency' or 'personal agency' to discriminate it from 'agencies' that provide services. However, in this book we just use the term agency.

Agency is about intentionally doing things, rather than allowing life to happen to you. Jeffery (2011:6) states that agency "implies the ability of individuals or groups to act on their situations, to behave as subjects rather than objects in their own lives, to shape their own circumstances and ultimately achieve change". Although the individual is seen as 'active', that is not to say that agency involves 'activity'. A person might decide not to do anything as a result of their awareness and choices and maintain the status quo. Acting within a rule, for example wearing a seat belt, might be because the person is complying, is using the rule as guidance, or is compelled to do so by law (Barnes, 2000: 47). These drivers will all motivate the same 'passive' seat belt wearing behaviour, but are very different expressions of agency. What is significant is that the individual is active in their own lives engaging with the events surrounding them (Barnes, 2000: 25).

A further important defining feature is that agency is not characterised by a successful outcome. Agency is being active in one's own life, regardless of how effective those actions might be (Paternoster and Pogarsky, 2009).

Bandura (2001: 3) describes how in order for people to make their way successfully through a complex world full of challenges and hazards, they have to make "good judgments about their capabilities, anticipate probable effects of different events and courses of action, size up sociocultural opportunities and constraints, and regulate behaviour accordingly". He states that this will "enable them to achieve desired outcomes and avoid unwanted ones". To achieve this complex task demands a range of skills or capabilities. We have categorised three key skills or capabilities: awareness, choice and action.

Awareness of self and of the structures that surround self (debated in the previous chapter) is vitally important as it expands choices. A limited view of the world leads to limited choice, whereas a wide view of the world provides wide choice. Parker (2000: 59) frames agents as needing "practical consciousness" drawn from their life experiences. Reflection on lived experiences is therefore necessary to develop such practical consciousness. This links with the experiential approach to learning described within critical pedagogy. For Edwards (2005), awareness incorporated 'know-what', 'know-how' and 'know-who' in her model of relational agency.

Choosing is a powerful act that involves reflection, conscious thought, judging the different merits of options and committing to an option in the form of a mental plan (Caldwell, 2006: 40). The act of choosing involves having an intention; a sense of a desired outcome. Bratman (2007: 21) has referred to this as reflectiveness and planfulness. Reflection informs choice as the person reviews what has made them happy or well and seeks other activities or outcomes that will satisfy that need. Reflection also informs the person as to what has previously been successful or unsuccessful, guiding the choice between different courses of action. Planning is a temporal activity (ibid, 28), in other words, it takes place over a period of time. The agent therefore needs to have a sense of time and will need to sequence actions over time to attempt to achieve the desired outcome. This might be in terms of minutes or weeks. This has implications for programmes that are time-bound and prescriptive. How can these afford the experiential approach of this type of self-discovery?

Acting on this plan and carrying it out is the final and perhaps most challenging aspect of agency (Bratman, 2007: 32). Many of us have made a mental plan to perhaps lose weight, but then failed to enact it. Enacting the plan therefore requires self-governance.

Agency involves the use of personal power and hence the significant underpinning of the next chapter on empowerment theory. Theorists on agency have defined power in terms of the power to choose (Parsons, 1937) and as the power to make a difference, to transform the structures and systems in which they are involved (Giddens, 1994). Archer's (2000: 162) agents were also bestowed with power. Archer described them developing 'personal emergent powers' through the process of socialisation, and it was these powers, she said, that enabled them to have agency.

Agency is also collective, rather than an individualistic model. People may individually have agency, but it is the collective expression of agency that shapes structures and the collectively constituted structures that enable and constrain individual agents. This is an important distinction that is attentive to the socially constructed nature of the world (Barnes, 2000: 54; Caldwell, 2006: 7). From a social constructivist stance, discourses construct social phenomena in different ways and so entail different possibilities for human actions. This clearly accounts for the ways in which structures are created and the ways in which agents engage in them (Burr, 1995:15). Such constructivist accounts are central to structure and agency and to the practice of critical pedagogy.

Our account of agency is deliberately practical. It describes how people develop awareness, choices and actions within social and cultural worlds. It is not a philosophical account of free will or determinism, but a functional social cultural model of behaviour. From this perspective, all CYPF need agency in order to successfully navigate life and all services that support them will seek to enhance their agency. The practitioners, managers and leaders that work with them also need agency to support them (Williams and Sullivan, 2009; Edwards, 2005). It is a concept applicable to all and a concept that can be translated into practical tools and activities.

Reflective activity

When have you felt like you have had a lot of agency at work or in your life? What were you aware of, what choices did you make, and what did you do?

Key theorists

As early as 1928, leading anthropologist Margaret Mead wrote that, "individuals need to be conceptualised as personally agentic, yet socially shaped over time". Yet, as we saw in the previous chapter, there were decades that saw sociologists denying human agency within the movement of structuralism. Over time, sociology came to bestow people with more agency. Weber (1978), for example, positioned agency within a societal context and introduced the possibility of an interplay between structure and agency. Weber's studies were limited, however, in that he adopted a focus that was exclusively at the meso level of structure. It only investigated status, religion, ideas and organisational structures and class (Weber, 1978). Whilst these were valuable moves towards understanding that people shaped discourses, there was a long way to go before people were seen as agents.

The first attempt to reconcile structure and agency was made by Bourdieu (1990). Bourdieu's (1998) concept of 'habitus' located individuals in social groups and social classes. Bourdieu saw different habitus competing to maintain their social standing in various settings. Individual agency was therefore shaped by the norms of the group, as the individuals within them sought inclusion within the habitus and sought to establish the superiority of that habitus. Strikingly, Bourdieu (1990) thought that habitus were developed collectively by generations of people in response to the experience of winning or losing as competitors in social fields. This acknowledges the socially con-structed nature of structures. A limitation of the notion of habitus is that 'competition' becomes the prime purpose of structure and agency (Parker, 2000: 48). This would not account for all behaviours.

Famously, in 1994, Anthony Giddens tackled the challenge of structure and agency head on, developing structuration theory. Rather than describing a dualism (structure versus agency), Giddens (1994: 9) describes a duality where objects and subjects are constitutive of each other. He described the structur-alist's position as 'objectivism', where structures are maintained without any reference to subjects. The agency perspective is the opposite of 'subjectivism', where agency operated without any reference to objects. His theoretical middle position sees objects and subjects relate to one another.

Giddens further argued that agency required understanding of dialogical con-texts and practical knowledge of the production and reproduction of social inter-action. Agency, for Giddens, was therefore dependent on being knowledgeable about a legacy of ways and means of doing things; it was innately social.

Archer deepened the argument that individuals and social structures are interdependent. Archer's view is sociocultural in the attention to the relation-ship between context, interaction and agents and to agents working together in social settings as 'corporate agents'.

Archer (2000) claims that structures pre-exist the agent, who is born into a predestined place of privilege (or non-privilege). This has huge implications when viewed alongside concepts of wellbeing and social justice, as those born into impoverished and oppressed settings immediately have less scope for agency. Archer goes on to describe an individual's 'involuntary situated' birth point as indicative of inequality. Further, "the circumstances in which we remain involuntarily embedded throughout childhood, condition what we project as possible, attainable and even desirable" (ibid: 262). This is a key difference to Giddens's model which was egalitarian.

This seems at odds with the central tenet of agency, about awareness, choice and action, as it indicated a predetermined life course and outcomes. However, Archer keeps the 'self' distinct from social interaction. In this way, Archer describes the agent as moving through the natural, practical and social realms of knowledge, co-acting, interacting and transacting, and developing personal emergent powers. Through socialisation individual agents act with others, becoming 'corporate agents' and having greater impact on the world shaping the structures into which others are born.

Although the complexity and language of Archer's work can be found to be inaccessible, it accounts for social in/justice through the pre-existence of structures that people are born into. It provides an account of the importance of socialisation in the development of 'power' supporting notions of social capital. Her model also shows how agents act on society individually and collectively reinforcing or changing structures. As such it is a strong model on which to base our ideas of structure, agency, wellbeing, social justice and critical pedagogy.

Structure and agency as a duality

In the previous chapter we discussed the nature of structures that act on people to either constrain or enable them to achieve what they want. In this chapter we have established that people have agency to act on those structures. The actions that people take, whether they are conforming to the structures or rebelling against them, will reinforce or change them. The norms of friendships, families, organisations, communities, countries and societies generally, are created by the actions of the people within them. Structures do not solely act on people, people also act on structures. This reciprocal relationship is known as a duality, where structure and agency exist together. As agency is dynamic and situational, a person's ability to act on or be acted on by structures will vary.

We conceptualise this relationship as a cycle. CYPF and those that work with them behave in certain ways and take certain actions. These actions and behaviours constitute their agency. The structures of society also act on them through norms of acceptable actions and behaviours, discourses that frame how they are perceived and laws that bind them. One does not exist without the other and the influence of one shapes the other. This is represented in Figure 6.1.

Even the largest structures, the macro structures, act in parallel with agency. The most obvious form of macro-level structures is policy. Policy is used by the government to 'legitimise' knowledge and meanings to the public (Bauman, 1989). Whilst the public are 'receivers' of such policy, they also hold power as they can choose to re-elect the government or not. The result is that the government needs to write policy that is broadly congruent with current norms of society, writing 'credible narratives' (Morrel, 2006: 371).

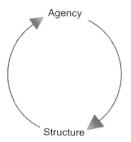

Figure 6.1 The structure agency duality

Thus policy shapes society and society confines policy. This is especially visible in the rise of consumer rights and service user consultation (Preston-Shoot, 2009: 9), as end-users are theoretically now able to directly shape public services, further increasing 'people' power.

Whilst policies exert power at a national level, they are open to influence. The policy is therefore rarely static, it is mediated by those that lead, manage and deliver it for a variety of reasons, such as a lack of belief in the policy, or its impracticability. Lipsky (1980: 141) refers to these people as actors or "street level bureaucrats". Mediation of policy is sometimes due to self-defence, and can be a coping mechanism in response to client demands and resource paucity (Nielson, 2006). The ideas communicated in policy are not always possible to implement in the complex shades of the real world and this also blocks its implementation (Frost, 2005: 6).

Agency, wellbeing and social justice

As we established in the introduction, we consider wellbeing and social justice to be in a relationship with one another. It is difficult for people to experience wellbeing in a situation that is socially unjust. Equally it is hard for people to contribute to social justice if they are not feeling good and functioning well (as per our definition of wellbeing).

With our new understanding of structure and agency we can see a reflection of the relationship between wellbeing and social justice. The extent to which a person experiences wellbeing is reflected by their agency. This view is supported by the literature on co-production (Coote, 2010) that presents services as most effective when co-produced with community members. It also resonates with the literature on the effect of personal control on wellbeing (Ledwith, 2011). The structures that enable or constrain their wellbeing are those of social justice.

With this in mind, we can now add structure and agency to our diagram of wellbeing and social justice (figure 6.2).

A family with a high level of awareness who makes choices and acts on them (i.e. has a high level of agency) is more likely to navigate the structures

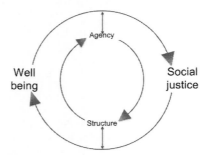

Figure 6.2 The relationship between structure and agency, wellbeing and social justice

of society successfully. If they choose to use their agency positively they are likely to experience enhanced wellbeing and can contribute to society to understand, challenge or support social justice. Equally a family who are oppressed with poverty may not experience wellbeing as they do not have their basic needs met. The unjust structures may compound their lack of wellbeing, for example, as they are not able to travel to find support or income. This detracts from their ability to choose an appropriate course of action (i.e. low agency).

We believe the strength of the relationship between these four key terms means that they cannot be treated individually. Working on one aspect of wellbeing, say obesity, will not be effective unless the person has the agency to choose healthy food most of the time. Healthy eating will not be sustainable if the person is living in poverty and unable to afford fresh fruit and vegetables. The constant advertising of fast foods and promotion of size zero women's bodies will undermine agency and wellbeing. These four terms are interwoven and need tackling together in order to achieve positive change for individuals, groups, communities, countries and the world.

Reflective activity

Think of a CYPF that you have worked with that demonstrated a high level of agency and a second one that demonstrated a low level of agency. Think about the following questions.

How did you know that they had high or low levels of agency?

What structures were they navigating and did these differ at all between the two?

How did their respective levels of agency affect their wellbeing?

In what ways were they subject to social in/justice?

How did they contribute to social in/justice?

What do you think the relationship is between structure, agency, wellbeing and social justice?

Benefits and limitations of an agentic perspective

There are many advantages of working from the perspective that CYPF have agency. The concept of agency is not fatalistic or deterministic and bestows hope to us all that we can be who or what we want to be, within reason. That reason is rendered comprehensible through understanding the structures that we can use to our advantage that enable our agency and those that work against us constraining our agency. The agentic perspective is founded on the belief that people can and do change their lives and can change structures rather than unconsciously and robotically reproducing them. The starting point of this process is awareness of the structures that we live within – a process that Freire (1972) described as critical consciousness. This is why a critical pedagogical approach is so allied to the agency perspective. If we believe in human agency then it follows that we believe that there is scope for social change. That if enough people will it, there will be increased wellbeing and social justice.

A limitation of the structure and agency debate is that it has been very academic and is in danger of remaining theoretical. Efforts must be made, as in this book, to make it a practical and useful concept. We need, as practitioners, to understand what we can do to reveal the enabling and constraining structures around us and what we can do to lever the agency of ourselves and those we support.

This is the rationale for the next chapter and part 2 of this book.

Vignette 6.1 Mark Johnson

As a young person Mark Johnson was subjected to extreme physical violence. He internalised the hatred of his father and became a drug addict:

> *No more hot tears for me. I won't cry again. Ever. My dad hates me and there's reason for that: I'm hateful. I hate myself. He despises me because I am despicable. I despise myself. Dad wants to destroy me because that's the best thing to do with kids like me. From now on I will destroy myself*
>
> Mark Johnson (2007: 84), reflecting on age 16.

Mark turned to drugs and alcohol in order to escape from the reality of his life, to destroy himself as his father had attempted to. At times he was violent himself perpetuating the pattern he experienced. He had a series of attempts to have relationships, to go 'straight'. But the self-destructive pattern prevailed. He was subjected to and recreated the structures he grew up in.

In later life Mark came very close to death, as his drug use and street life had become so perilous. In time, he realised that he had to turn things around; that he would not survive if he continued life as he was. He joined a drug rehabilitation programme. He got 'straight':

> *I reached a point where there were two options for me. To accept help and listen to others who had gone through it before me. Or to die. It may seem obvious, but it wasn't to me then and it took me a long time to make the right choice* (ibid: 340).

Mark set up his own business with funding from the Prince's Trust and years after success, now helps other young people to rehabilitate. He has been awarded the *Daily Mirror*'s Pride of Britain Award. He states that this validation, and the new purpose that he has found in life, have given him a better high than drugs ever did:

> *I've been given the greatest of gifts: the chance to help others the way I was helped. No drink or drugs ever made me feel so good. And in this lies the solution to my problem* (ibid: 340).

There are many turning points in Mark's story. There are many people who helped him. Sean, for example, "saved him". Sean got Mark into Turning Point – a rehabilitation centre in London. When Mark relapsed and used, he should have been thrown out of the centre. Mark realises this and yet is honest with Sean, pleading with him to help, knowing that either the drugs or the people on the street will kill him if he is thrown out. Sean trusts in Mark, bends the rules and finds Mark a new rehabilitation centre away from London.

Although not the final step in Mark's journey, this was the first significant investment of time, energy and trust between Mark and Sean. Mark was ready to be helped, but unable to be helped in the given circumstances. Sean was ready to help, even against the rules and against the odds. This highlights two key points that we will return to in the following chapter: the need for a 'spark' to initiate empowerment and the need for sustained support, despite recycling to earlier behaviours.

Summary of key points

Agency is the ability to be aware, choose and act. Everyone has and uses agency, but to varying degrees depending on time and context. Using our agency may not necessarily create positive outcomes as we may use it to negative ill intent, or our good intentions may not come to fruition. Agency, therefore, cannot be measured by outcome. Agency is affected by and affects structures. They exist in a mutually reinforcing duality.

We believe that CYPF can be supported to use their agency to experience enhanced wellbeing and social justice. We also believe that we, practitioners, can use our agency to support our own and others' wellbeing and social justice. To do this we need to become aware of the structures that surround us. Just as social justice and wellbeing work in relationship with one another, so do structures and agency. Enhanced agency and the levering of enabling structures increase opportunity for wellbeing and social justice. This is true for individuals, groups and communities of CYPF. Structure, agency, wellbeing and social justice are therefore in a relationship with one another.

The process of empowerment levers the state of agency and therefore wellbeing and social justice. This is the focus of the next chapter.

Further reading

Barnes, B. (2000). *Understanding Agency: Social Theory and Responsible Action*. London: Sage.

Bauman, Z. (1989). *Legislators and Interpreters*. Oxford: Polity Press.
Caldwell, R. (2006). *Agency and Change*. Abingdon: Routledge.
Jeffery, L. (2011). *Understanding Agency Social Welfare and Change*. Bristol: Policy Press. This book is very accessible and offers a clear account of structure and agency in the context of social work in the UK.
Johnson, M. (2007) *Wasted*. St Ives: Sphere Books.

References

Archer, M. (2000). *Being Human, the problem of agency*. Cambridge: Cambridge University Press.
Bandura, A. (2001). 'Social Cognitive Theory: An Agentic Perspective', *Annual Review of Psychology*, 52(1), pp. 1–26.
Barnes, B. (2000). *Understanding Agency: Social Theory and Responsible Action*. London: Sage.
Bauman, Z. (1989). *Legislators and Interpreters*. Oxford: Polity Press.
Bourdieu, P. (1990). *The Logic of Practice*. Translated by R. Nice. Cambridge: Polity Press.
Bourdieu, P. (1998). *Practical Reason: On the Theory of Action*. Cambridge: Polity Press.
Bratman, M. E. (2007). *Structures of Agency*. Oxford: Oxford University Press.
Burr, V. (1995). *An Introduction to Social Constructionism*. London: Routledge.
Caldwell, R. (2006). *Agency and Change*. Abingdon: Routledge.
Coote, A. (2010). *Ten Big Questions about the Big Society and Ten Ways to Make the Best of It*. London: nef.
Edwards, A. (2005). 'Relational Agency: Learning to be a Resourceful Practitioner', *International Journal of Educational Research*, 43, pp. 168–182.
Freire, P. (1970). *Pedagogy of the Oppressed*. London: Continuum Publishing Company.
Freire, P. (1972).*Cultural Action for Freedom*. London: Penguin.
Frost, N. (2005). *Professionalism, Partnership and Joined-up Thinking: A Research Review of Front-line Working with Children and Families*. Totnes: Research in Practice.
Giddens, A. (1994). *Beyond the Left and the Right, the Future of Radical Politics*. Cambridge: Polity Press.
Jeffery, L. (2011). *Understanding Agency Social Welfare and Change*. Bristol: Policy Press.
Johnson, M. (2007). *Wasted*. St Ives: Sphere Books.
Ledwith, M. (2007). Reclaiming the radical agenda: A critical approach to community development. Concept, 17(2), 8–12. Reproduced in *The Encyclopaedia of Informal Education*. Retrieved 1st January 2011 from: www.infed.org/community/critical_community_development.htm
Ledwith, M.(2011).*Community Development: A Critical Approach*, 2ndedn.London: Polity Press.
Lipsky, M. (1980). *Street Level Bureaucracy: Dilemmas of the Individual in Public Services*. New York: Russell Sage Foundation.
Mead, M. (1928). *Coming of Age in Samoa: A Psychological Study of Primitive Youth for Western Civilisation*. New York: Harper Collins.

Morrel, K. (2006). 'Policy as Narrative in New Labour's Reform of the NHS', *Public Administration Review*, 84(2), pp. 367–385.

Nielson, V. (2006). 'Are Street Level Bureaucrats Compelled or Enticed to Cope?', *Public Administration Review*, 84(4), pp. 861–889.

Parker, J. (2000). *Structuration*. Oxford University Press: Buckingham.

Parsons, T. (1937). *The Structure of Social Action*. Maidenhead: McGraw Hill.

Paternoster, R. and Pogarsky, G. (2009). 'Rational Choice, Agency, and Thoughtfully Reflective Decision Making: The Short and Long-term Consequences of Making Good Choices', *School of Criminal Justice*, 25, pp. 103–127.

Preston-Shoot, M. (2009). 'Repeating History? Observations on the Development of Law and Policy for Integrated Practice', in McKimm, J., and Phillips, K. (eds) *Leadership and Management of Integrated Services*. Poole: Learning Matters, pp. 35–56.

Weber, M. (1978). *Economy and Society*. Berkeley, CA: University of California Press.

Williams, P., and Sullivan, H. (2009). 'Faces of Integration', *International Journal of Integrated Care*, 9, 1–13.

7 Wellbeing, empowerment and oppression

Chapter overview

Empowerment is a process where individuals and groups develop agency, countering oppression, towards social justice and wellbeing. Empowerment is not something that can be 'gifted' to or 'bestowed' on people. We cannot 'do it' to other people, yet this is often how the word 'empowerment' is used in policy and practice. This chapter provides an empowerment framework for practice. It breaks down key elements of the process of empowerment and how we can use this in our practice to support CYPF to develop agency towards social justice and more sustainable wellbeing.

What is empowerment?

Broadly, empowerment can be seen as "people taking control of their lives" (Kohn, 1991: 7) and "becoming a leader in your own life" (Galland, 1980 in Angell, 1994: 96). It is about people gaining greater control of their lives and circumstances (Thompson, 2007).

Of most significance is exploring what 'power' means in empowerment. Gutierrez (1990) described empowerment as "a process of increasing personal, interpersonal, or political power so that individuals, families or communities can take action to improve their circumstances" (p. 149). This refers to empowerment as a process. By claiming our personal power, we are able to have control over our lives.

Control is also a key dimension of empowerment and indeed an outcome of practice that supports empowerment. Adams (2008: 17) describes both the process and outcome of empowerment, suggesting:

> The capacity of individuals, groups and communities to take control of their circumstances, exercise power and achieve their own goals, and the process by which, individually and collectively, they are able to help themselves and others to maximize the quality of their lives.

Zimmerman (2000) described empowerment as comprising three factors: intrapersonal, interactional and behavioural (Sibthorp and Arthur-Banning, 2004). The **intrapersonal** component included internal factors that influence a person's perception of their empowerment, such as motivation, self-efficacy, perceived competence and an internal locus of control (perceived control). The **interactional** factor included a person's interaction within given environmental constraints, whilst the **behavioural** factors included the actions required to achieve outcomes (Sibthorp and Arthur-Banning, 2004). To experience empowerment, CYPF would therefore need to have self-esteem, motivation, self-efficacy, an internal locus of control and behavioural options, within a given environment. Zimmerman's ideas have started to unpack the complexity of a term that is often used in oversimplified ways.

Empowerment is not a fixed state – this lends additional complexity. How empowered people feel will vary from time to time, and situation to situation. A young person may feel empowered to talk in front of his or her peer group, but not in front of adults or vice versa. The same young person's sense of empowerment may vary day to day in both those situations depending on how well they feel. Empowerment is therefore both dynamic and situational.

What empowerment isn't!

We hear the term empowerment with increasing regularity, within practice, mission statements and policy. Although we are delighted to hear the term, we also feel the need to raise caution to how the term is being used. Empowerment has become something of a buzzword in recent years; a term that is sprayed around to make projects appealing and perhaps speaking to policy that has alluded to empowerment (Huebner, 1998; Ledwith, 2011; Mullender *et al.*, 2013).

Empowerment is an intrinsic process; it comes from within – be this individually, in families or in communities. As such, it cannot be given to someone and therefore we cannot empower CYPF. As soon as we suggest this, we are stating our power over them and that power is ours to gift. Our projects don't empower people; they provide catalytic conditions for CYPF to become empowered. In chapter 4, we similarly challenged policy such as the Big Society, which talked of 'empowering people' and 'giving them power'. Empowerment is not an attribute or skill that can be packaged and passed over. Ledwith (2011) criticised this policy for being strong on the rhetoric of empowerment and weak on equality.

Vignette 7.1 The National Citizen Service

The National Citizen Service was announced as the flagship initiative of the Big Society (Cabinet Office, 2010b). This aimed to increase the civic responsibility of young people by introducing a community action project. St Croix (2011: 52) highlights the disempowering nature of the development of this policy – a closed house process of the privileged few, excluding young people and practitioners, and encoded in a discourse that marginalises youth work. Further, the programme itself does not seem to have empowered young people – as five per cent of young people were dismissed from the Challenge Trust trial schemes because of misbehaviour (Natasha, 2010 in St Croix, 2011).

It would seem, therefore, that the Big Society is actually quite a small and elite society after all.

The co-opting of the language of empowerment places it at risk of corruption. The term can be exploited when people are 'selected' for consultations, risking tokenism. Does what they say have any weight, or has it already been decided? When service users are involved in how to spend their personalised budget, are they empowered or simply being pacified in decision making about depleted resources? Are service users participating in the reinforcement of other people's agendas rather than their own? Are any of these practices authentic in their empowerment, if we are not asking people to question the structures within which they are set. The process of empowerment therefore demands a high level of critical pedagogy to avoid working on a superficial level or reinforcement of existing dominant structures and benignly reinforcing oppression.

Disempowerment

To further support our thinking, it is worthwhile noting the opposite of empowerment – disempowerment. Taking people's power away from them occurs through the processes of oppression, discrimination and marginalisation. Disempowerment is to deprive of power, authority or influence, to make weak, ineffectual or unimportant. Just as we discuss empowerment as a process, disempowerment can be seen as the vehicle of oppression.

Oppression is often on the basis of difference. In chapter 5 we introduced 'othering' as the process of defining people as 'other' than ourselves (Jensen, 2011). It can be tempting to portray oneself as OK, and everyone else as different or 'other'. This process enables us to stay safe. Over there 'they' get addicted to drugs, but that is because they are different and other than us. We are therefore safe and insulated from the risk of addiction. Once people have been construed as 'other', it is then simple to also treat them as abject (Tyler, 2013). By treating sex workers as abject, 'disgusting and disgraceful', we, the respectable, are able to turn a blind eye to their oppression. By treating recipients of welfare benefits as 'scroungers', we can avoid our culpability in their poverty. In effect, othering and social abjection are dehumanising. The process dehumanises the victims and the oppressors (Freire, 1970).

These terms can therefore become important test benches for our practice. For example, a project that automatically excludes young people who are badly behaved can be seen as oppressive, power laden, reinforcing the sense that adults are powerful and young people are powerless, discriminating against them on the basis of their actions and marginalising them out of the project and onto the streets. In contrast, a project that used young people's disruptive behaviour as a topic of conversation and worked through it with the young people, asking them for ways ahead and solutions, can be seen as empowering. It disrupts the normal power relations and communicates that everyone has an equal right to make decisions about group behaviours.

As empowerment is a personal sense of power, we are therefore careful to talk about practice that is empowering. Careful that the focus is on creating conditions in which CYPF can claim their power. This can make empowering practice problematic for practitioners. Whilst we may teach a child to read in a step-by-step logical way, developing skills progressively, there is no core set of skills that comprise empowerment. It is a complex state, a feeling or sense. The challenge for practitioners is therefore to create an environment for CYPF to develop power. The process of empowerment below provides a road map for the creation of those conditions.

The process of empowerment

The reactive self

Campbell and MacPhail (2002) suggested that most empowerment work starts with the assumption that there is powerlessness or lack of control over destiny. We therefore can assume that empowerment comes from a dis-empowered place. This is defined in the model of empowerment (Figure 7.1) as a **reactive** place. CYPF may be reacting to the world in which they find themselves because they not only lack control, but they do not know what other options there are. They are going with the flow and are stuck in the status quo. For many CYPF this is a world of chaotic family situations, a feeling of a lack of love and security, disengagement from education that has failed to capture their interest, external pressure from peers and society and disconnection from what we and they might come to know as positive trajectories.

Many CYPF do not describe or recognise themselves as disempowered or oppressed. They may, however, demonstrate powerlessness to us even though they do not see it in themselves. There may be little reference to powerlessness whilst powerless and critically unaware. This only becomes apparent to them once they have recognised that there are other ways of being and thus people may only recognise their disempowerment once empowered. For example, a sexually exploited young woman may not recognise herself as sexual exploited or disempowered when we first start working with her. Freire (1973) defined this as where people are naïve rather than critically conscious (discussed in chapter 4). At this stage, people lack insight into the way in which their social conditions undermine their wellbeing and so do not see their own actions as capable of changing these conditions (Campbell and MacPhail, 2002).

Freire argued that people need to become aware of their own oppression before they can do anything about changing it. However, we argue that CYPF cannot be told this. Being told is more likely to lead to pushing back against the teller. Many of us are guilty of saying *"stop hanging around with them; they're no good for you"*, but this must be realised not told. Thus, our role is to create time and space to discover they have control and power, there are other options and they are capable (they have agency). This inadvertently can reveal powerlessness to young people. This can be traumatic, however should not be thought of as 'opening a can of worms', but becoming critically conscious.

With time and space comes the opportunity for the discovery of self. An increased self-awareness is underpinned by the concept of raising critical consciousness. This can be seen by understanding an individual's journey through gaining awareness of their power (or lack of); learning to question, rather than simply accept the status quo; leading to insight into other opportunities and ways of being, and their potential to change their circumstance (Robins *et al.*, 1998). Increased self-awareness and thus critical consciousness, is depicted in the empowerment model as three levels: Sparking, Realising and Wanting. Each of these is considered below.

Reflective activity

Do you recognise CYPF you have worked with as reacting to the world around them?
What behaviours did they display?
How did you work with them?

Sparking

Coleman (2007) identified the need to provide positive experiences to 'interrupt' the chain reaction of negative events. This in turn is a catalyst, sparking a different chain of events. Similarly, Henderson *et al.* (2007) worked with the concept of 'critical moments'. They drew from Denzin's (1989) discussion of 'epiphanies', Mandlebaum's (1973) discussion of 'turning points', Humphrey's (1993) discussion of 'breaks', and Giddens's (1991) discussion of 'fateful moments'. Giddens (1991: 143) defined these moments as "times when events come together in such a way that an individual stands at a crossroads in their existence or where a person learns of information with fateful consequences". Henderson et al. state that these fateful moments can potentially be empowering experiences.

These sparking moments can be either positive or negative. Hart (1996) suggested that new experiences or special challenges often served to spark the empowerment process. Whereas Gutierrez (1994) proposed that stressful life events could also catalyse the empowerment process. Both of these perspectives are represented by the positive and negative sparking in the model. As practitioners, we see on a daily basis sparking from positive events, such as being away on residential, a sense of achievement, or being listened to for seemingly the first time. We therefore need to focus on sparking activities that are catalytic. We can create these sparks with our approach to practice – our critical pedagogy. Our equity, our listening and not telling, and our questioning, provide a different perspective to the disempowered or oppressed. We also see sparking come about from negative events, such as an assault or an arrest. Be the catalyst positive or negative, it leads to a state of realising something different to what has come before.

Realising

Sparking activities are perhaps most powerful when combined with a period of reflection. Asking CYPF to reflect on critical questions at this heightened time can pave a path for them to begin to make connections and realisations. Becker (2008) sees this point as crisis, as it is asking them to question what they have come to know as the truth previously. He states that "In the crisis the individuals are confronted with themselves. They learn something about themselves ... Thus the crisis turns into a kind of self-enlightenment" (ibid: 11).

From a youth work and informal learning perspective, Batsleer (2008: 6) referred to a need for recognition of learning which involved,

> watching for 'the penny to drop' and listening for signs of 'moving on' [as] a significant element of practice. Youth workers look out for these moments in the conversation, as it develops, when something clicks, when something has been achieved so that learning is acknowledged and recognised.

Gibson (1995) similarly referred to a phase of 'discovering reality'. This may be realising a heightened sense of one's self and/or situation, which leads to an awareness. Summerson Carr (2003) suggested that this was a process of creating identity not simply discovering it from history. It was not a static, fixed or attainable notion of identity to be rediscovered, but an on-going process, changeable and full of potential (de Lauretis, 1986). Zimmerman (1990: 72) suggests that "experiences that provide opportunities to enhance perceived control will help individuals cope with stress and solve problems in their personal lives". Similarly, Friedli (1997) described the importance of giving CYPF opportunities to take control of their own life.

Our work with CYPF therefore needs to provide opportunities to explore and enhance perceived control, so they become aware of the control they can have in their lives, as well as developing and practising being in control and making choices and decisions.

Taniguchi *et al.* (2005) refer to this process as potentially painful. 'Realising' can mean being overwhelmed by the discovery of true self and thus may not be a pleasurable experience. This is also known as cognitive dissonance (Cooper, 1990), in which there is discomfort in having two contrasting ideas simultaneously (e.g. I can do what I want, and I can't do anything). This can further be experienced through realising perceived empowerment rather than actual, in which they may experience a 'reality dip'.

Wanting

Summerson Carr (2003) suggests that opening up a range of possibilities about who one can be and how one can act, inspires mobilisation for change. This is characterised in the model by realising what you want. This is a wanting of change, difference, or something more specific such as getting a job. This is an intrinsic motivation, in that it comes from within the participant, from the realisations they make, rather than something they are told to do or imposed upon them and which they may have previously pushed away or fought. Parpart *et al.* (2003) referred to this phase as strengthening the 'power within'.

Arneson (1999) made an important critique to using the term 'wanting', arguing that something can intrinsically enhance an individual's wellbeing even though they might hate it. It is often hard to make some of the realisations that CYPF do. However, the effect is that they become more critically conscious and have a better understanding of what is good or bad for them. Ultimately, this is a step towards a more enhanced wellbeing: more critically conscious of your well-ness or lack thereof. This results in a knowing and in a desire for specific actions and pathways. Therefore, 'wanting' is not simply desire fulfilment, but a raised critical consciousness that leads to knowledge and aspirations that contribute to enhancing one's own wellbeing. Desire fulfilment alone may not contribute to wellbeing, as it is temporary and ultimately can be damaging to wellbeing.

Reflective activity

Have you ever ignored what someone has told you time and time again, only to later come to the same conclusion about it yourself?
How did you respond to being told?
How did it feel to come to this conclusion yourself?

Proactive commitment

An intrinsic motivation for change can initiate proactive commitments, illuminating a distinct shift from the previous reactive state. This is a commitment to action and marks the mobilisation for change (Friedmann, 1992). This is a significant point, as it distinguishes action from reflection; active

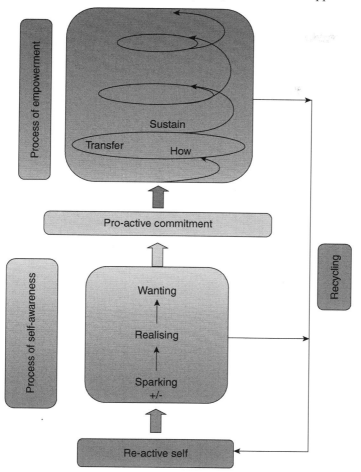

Figure 7.1 The framework of empowerment (Maynard, 2011: 273).

from passive; from realising and wanting something, to doing something about it. Freire (1973), amongst other authors (e.g. Friedmann, 1992), identified a similar 'turning point' (Hur, 2006), 'tipping point' (Gladwell, 2000), or 'maximising step' (Hur, 2006).

Mobilisation into action can be thought of as an awakening to the personal becoming political. Cox (1991) stated that through the process of critical interpretation, new understandings arise that provide the basis for personal and social transformation. Forming new understandings of one's position brings about a commitment to do something about it (showing internal locus of control). Hur (2006: 530) poignantly summarised, "at this point, empowerment reaches the point that the people feel able to utilise their confidence, desires, and abilities to bring about 'real change'".

Learning how

Within this proactive process, people seek answers to their own questions. They develop belief in their ability (self-efficacy) to be different and seek out new skills. At this point, as facilitators of this process, we also become a resource for CYPF to draw information from, through suggestion or signposting. However, this is only once this point has been reached intrinsically. If we input before this, we run the risk of being interpreted as 'telling' CYPF what to do.

At this stage, we can introduce more tools and strategies for CYPF to utilise in their forward momentum. For example, if people acknowledge anger as a barrier for them, we can introduce activities directly related to anger management.

Transfer of learning

As CYPF start to think about how they can implement the changes they have started to make, we need to consider how we facilitate the transfer of learning from one context to another. For example, they may make realisations and commit to changes on a programme with us, but what is crucial is how this is able to be transferred and implemented in different aspects of their lives. Research has shown that benefits gained from projects supporting CYPF have been transferred to the daily lives of participants (Holman and McAvoy, 2005). Luckner and Nadler (1997) state that the generalisation of learning was the application of what people learned as a result of attending an experiential course. This, they continued, occurred when the learning in one situation carried over to another. Similarly, Williamson and Taylor (2005) suggested that processing experiences helped people to bring a structured experience and different settings or experiences closer together. Optimally, they stated, these experiences become interwoven so that the awareness and growth that occurred during the experiential learning programme produced gains for use in other settings and situations.

As facilitators of the empowerment process, we need to make sure we help people transfer learning beyond their time with us. We need to make this explicit and allow people time to explore how they will feel being critically conscious in an environment that may not change.

Sustaining

Ryan and Deci (2000) stated that comparisons between people whose motivation was authentic (literally, self-authored or endorsed) had more interest, excitement and confidence than those who were externally controlled for an action (because they have been told to by another, law, or policy). This manifests in enhanced performance, persistence and creativity, as well as heightened vitality, self-esteem and general wellbeing. Persistence in particular is crucial for CYPF to be resilient to external disabling structures and fight for what they want. Schoon and Bynner (2003) identified resilience as the capacity of human beings to overcome adversity and to show positive adaptation in the face of that adversity. Thus, resilience is the ability to 'bounce back', or 'bounce forward' in the face of adversity and positive adaptation to competently create lives in which the individual has control. Crucial within this is challenging the adversity and not accepting it as socially just.

Related to resilience is the concept of 'flourishing'. Both concepts have been developed through the work of positive psychology. Fredrichson and Losada (2005) stated that to flourish meant to live within an optimal range of human functioning; one that connotes goodness, generativity, growth and resilience. It follows that, an individual who develops an ability to optimally function, in their worlds, is likely to show more sustained empowerment; upwardly spiralling and growing.

An empowered person could be seen to cope with different challenges in their life by transferring skills learnt from previous experiences to problem solve and come up with solutions to those challenges, thus sustaining an empowered cycle. The cycle of sustained empowerment within Figure 7.1, shows empowerment upwardly spiralling, pro-active, problem solving and flourishing for longer periods of time. This also characterised upwardly spiralling social mobility and ultimately characterises CYPF agency.

Hur (2006) states that maximised empowerment could be practised at the final stage of empowerment to overcome social oppression and achieve social justice. However, to use the word 'final' is not realistic, as empowerment is an on-going process, not a final destination. Moreover, often CYPF can recycle around to a reactive place.

Recycling

Ryan and Deci (2000) suggested that despite humans being liberally endowed with intrinsic motivational tendencies, evidence exists that the maintenance and enhancement of this inherent propensity required supportive conditions and networks, as it could be disrupted by various non-supportive conditions or networks. Non-supportive conditions are social environments that are antagonistic towards positive developmental tendencies. This links to the discussion of structures in chapter 5 and can be seen to enable or constrain transfer of learning and sustainable commitments and change.

It is common to see a drop-off after programmes, where participants return to old behaviours or are unable to reach or sustain commitments. Leberman and Martin (2004) describe a post-course 'fade-out effect' which could adversely affect transfer (Hattie *et al.*, 1997; Beard and Wilson, 2002).

The Transtheoretical Model of behaviour change (Prochaska and DiClemente, 1984) offers some theoretical underpinning to understanding this unsustainability. The authors suggest that most people would 'relapse' to previous stages before successful behaviour change was achieved (Prochaska *et al.*, 1992; Sarkin *et al.*, 2001). Sutton (1996) states that it is likely that individuals will relapse and typically cycle through the stages several times before achieving long-term maintenance or change.

We suggest that if this is likely, we should plan for it and actually see it as an experiential process and therefore positive. Thus, we refer to this as 'recycling', rather than relapse or regression. As facilitators we can make this explicit and worked towards through activities that can raise awareness of the pressures of social networks, for example. We also need to provide on-going opportunities to spark the recycling through the empowerment process again, in realising themselves to have recycled to a reactive place.

We are all susceptible to becoming reactive in the world and feeling out of control. Thus, to recycle through the process of empowerment is crucial to more sustainable empowerment. Individuals can gain greatly by learning from their disempowerment having previously been critically conscious as they could tune in to more specific details and strengthen their commitment to action. This can be experienced negatively, particularly the frustration that can be felt by a disempowered-empowered person.

Brown (2015: 37) describes this as "rising strong" from setbacks and "face hurt in a way that brings more wisdom and wholeheartedness to our lives". This challenges the true awareness we have of our situations and the assumptions of what truth is, what self-protection is and what needs to change if we want to lead more wholehearted lives. This encourages writing a new chapter to our story, based on the key learning and using this new braver story to change how we engage with the world and ultimately transform it. This acknowledges the pain and hurt of recycling and transforms it into an opportunity for learning, so that we recycle back to a stronger place than we were before.

Reflective activity

Look back at the model and see if you can recognise CYPF progression through the process of empowerment.

What would be the most helpful practitioner response to CYPF recycling – and why is that?

Collective action

Proactive people are problem solvers who are open to exploring how to make changes. They are also more open to feedback regarding their behaviour and to employing tools to change this. Within much of our practice, this occurs in a group work. The empowerment process is, for some, enhanced when shared with peers. Sharing and listening to each other can also be empowering. This is the personal becoming collective, as together they may realise their oppression. Sharing stories is a powerful tool for collective action. Ledwith (2011: 62) referred to this as "collective narratives for change". Ledwith suggests that autonomy and action gather strength in a collective process:

the simple act of listening to people's stories, respectfully giving one's full attention, is an act of personal empowerment, but to bring about change for social justice this process needs to be collective and needs to be located within wider structures.

We can see clear steps to social justice for wellbeing: individual readiness; group value and support; and collective action. Ledwith further states that "personal empowerment through a process of raising critical consciousness is the beginning stage of collective action for transformative change" (p. 97). Parpart *et al.* (2003) similarly referred to this as seeking out support groups and positive allies.

It is powerful to experience critical consciousness collectively and this is the foundation of collection action for change in communities; united not only in their knowledge that life can be different, but also in their desire to make change. This is an explicit process and although some of our work may be in groups, this does not necessarily mean it is facilitating collective action. To follow through to its collective potential, practice needs to offer critical insight for action. This asserts that simple self-awareness alone will not fulfil collective action and thus is not empowering in itself.

Linking empowerment and agency

This process of empowerment details how people with perceived agency or no agency claim their own power – their self-esteem, self-efficacy and an internal locus of control, as well as the skills and knowledge that they need at that particular time. Empowerment is a transformative process, gaining "transformative capacity" (Giddens, 1984: 15). The empowerment process levers agency – the more empowered, the more agentic the individual or group. This means that they have more awareness of themselves and the world around them, more awareness of choices, more ability to make a choice, and the ability to enact the choice behaviourally.

As discussed in chapter 6, agency interacts with structure. Structures therefore enable or constrain the process of empowerment. This is the situational nature of empowerment in action. On occasions, the structures in the world at any given point may overwhelm an individual leaving them disempowered and unable to enact their agency – and vice versa. The links between the process of empowerment and structure and agency is captured in Figure 7.2 below. The boundary of structures surrounds the process of empowerment and acts in relationship with agency.

Linking empowerment, agency, structure, wellbeing and social justice

This process of empowerment provides the detail leading to agency that was captured in chapter 6 as awareness-choice-action. The framework for developing awareness, choice and action is therefore at the heart of our model,

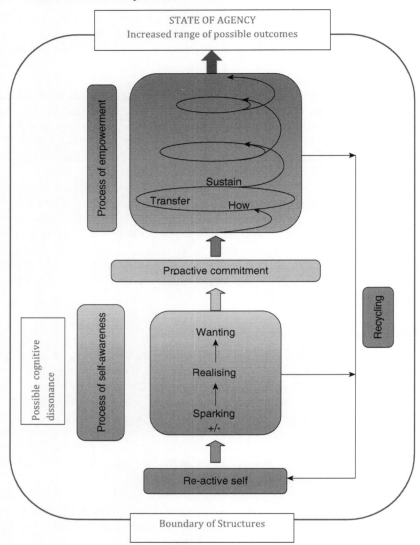

Figure 7.2 The link between empowerment and agency

depicted in Figure 7.3. The chapters of this book have built this model: the relationship of social justice and wellbeing, of structure and agency and of the empowerment process at the heart of it.

Chapter 1 detailed how social justice and wellbeing interact with one another. The more socially just the world is, the more CYPF will experience high levels of wellbeing. Conversely, in a world where a high number of CYPF experience high levels of wellbeing, there is likely to be more social justice.

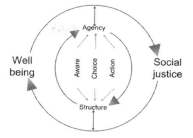

Figure 7.3 The Wellbeing and Social Justice Model

The structures that CYPF live in will offer varying degrees of equality and equity; they will be socially just or unjust. Their agency therefore operates on social justice by operating on the structures of the world. Social justice and its expression in structures will enable and constrain the agency of CYPF in socially just or unjust ways. Structure and agency are therefore connected reciprocally to social justice.

Equally the structures that CYPF live in will enable or constrain wellbeing. These structures will affect how well CYPF feel and how they function. CYPF may also use their agency to develop their wellbeing, engaging in actions that help them to thrive. Conversely CYPF may be so unwell and function in such a way that their agency is hindered. Structures and agency therefore also have a reciprocal relationship with wellbeing.

Critical pedagogy is the approach, and empowerment the process that supports CYPF agency within the structures that they live in (Alsop and Heinsohn, 2005: 6).

When we place these concepts together, we build a model of wellbeing and social justice that also locates structure and agency and the role of critical pedagogy and the process of empowerment.

Summary of key points

Empowerment has been misused as a buzzword and has been conceptually exploited, professionalised and colonised. Empowerment is a complex concept that involves developing self-esteem, self-efficacy and an internal locus of control. It is also a dynamic and situational state. Empowerment cannot be 'given' to CYPF, they must develop it for themselves. Therefore, practitioners create catalytic conditions in which CYPF may empower themselves. The process of empowerment presented in this chapter can be used as a framework for practice to support empowerment. The process of empowerment sits within critical pedagogy, as the key approach to support wellbeing. As such it is central to young people's navigation of structures and agency and will support wellbeing and social justice.

Further reading

Gutierrez, L. (1994). 'Beyond Coping: An Empowerment Perspective on Stressful Life Events', *Journal of Sociology and Social Welfare*, 21, 201–219.
Huebner, A. J. (1998). 'Examining "Empowerment": A How-to Guide for the Youth Development Professional', *Journal of Extension*, 36(6).
Parpart, J. L., Rai, S. M., and Standt, K. (2003). *Rethinking Empowerment: Gender and Development in a Global/Local World*. New York: Routledge.
Summerson Carr, S. (2003). 'Rethinking Empowerment Theory Using a Feminist Lens: The Importance of Process', *Affilia*, 18(1), 8–20.
Thompson, N. (2007). *Power and Empowerment*. Lyme Regis: Russell House Publishing.

References

Adams, R. (2008). *Empowerment, Participation and Social Work*. 4th edn. Basingstoke: Palgrave Macmillan.
Alsop, R., and Heinsohn, N. (2005). *Measuring Empowerment in Practice: Structuring Analysis and Framing Indicators*. World Bank Research Working Paper. World Bank.
Angell, J. (1994). 'The Wilderness Solo: An Empowering Growth Experience for Women', in Cole, E., Erdman, E., and Rothblum, E. D. (eds.), *Wilderness Therapy for Women: The Power of Adventure*. New York: Harrington Park Press, pp. 85–99.
Arneson, R. J. (1999). 'Human Flourishing Versus Desire Satisfaction', *Social Philosophy & Policy*, 16, 113–142.
Batsleer, J. (2008). *Informal Learning in Youth Work*. London: Sage Publications.
Beard, C., and Wilson, J. P. (2002). *The Power of Experiential Learning – A Handbook for Trainers and Educators*. London, UK: Kogan Page.
Becker, P. (2008). '*Outdoor practices and outdoor equipment – fields and spaces to form, to test and to present different forms of (bourgeois) subjectivity*'. Paper presented at the International mountain and outdoor conference, (November), Hruba Skala.
Brown, B. (2015). *Rising Strong*. San Francisco: Vermillion.
Cabinet Office (2010a). *Building the Big Society*. London: Cabinet Office.
Cabinet Office (2010b). *National Citizenship Service*. London: Cabinet Office.
Campbell, C. and MacPhail, C. (2002). 'Peer Education, Gender and the Development of Critical Consciousness: Participatory HIV Prevention by South African Youth', *Social Science and Medicine*, 55(2), 331–345.
Coleman, J. (2007). 'Emotional Health and Well Being', in Coleman, J., Hendry, L. and Kelop, M. (eds.), *Adolescence and Health*. London: John Wiley, pp. 41–60.
Cooper, J. (1990). *Cognitive Dissonance, 50 Years of a Classic Theory*. London: Sage.
Cox, E. O. (1991). 'The Critical Role of Social Action in Empowerment Orientated Groups', *Social Work With Groups*, 14, 77–90.
de Lauretis, T. (1986). 'Introduction', in de Lauretis, T. (ed.), *Feminist Studies/Critical Studies*. Bloomington: Indiana University Press, pp. 1–19.
Denzin, N. K. (1989). *Interpretive Biography*, Qualitative Research Methods Series, No. 17. London: Sage Publications.
Fredrichson, B. L., and Losada, M. F. (2005). 'Positive Affect and the Complex Dynamics of Human Flourishing', *American Psychologist*, 60(7), 678–686.
Freire, P. (1970). *Pedagogy of the Oppressed*. Harmondsworth: Penguin.

Freire, P. (1973). *Education for a Critical Consciousness*. New York: Seabury Press.

Friedli, L. (1997). *Mental Health Promotion: A Quality Framework*. London: Mental Health Foundation.

Friedmann, J. (1992). *Empowerment: Politics of Alternative Development*. Malden, MA: Blackwell Publishers.

Gibson, C. H. (1995). 'The Process of Empowerment in Mothers of Chronically Ill Children', *Journal of Advanced Nursing*, 21(6), 1201–1210.

Giddens, A. (1991). *Modernity and Self Identity: Self and Society in the Late Modern Age*. Cambridge: Polity.

Giddens, A. (1994). *Beyond the Left and the Right, the Future of Radical Politics*. Cambridge: Polity Press.

Gladwell, M. (2000). *The Tipping Point: How Little Things Can Make a Big Difference*. New York: Little, Brown and Company.

Gutierrez, L. (1990). 'Working with Women of Color: An Empowerment Perspective', *Social Work*, 35 (2), 149–153.

Gutierrez, L. (1994). 'Beyond Coping: An Empowerment Perspective on Stressful Life Events', *Journal of Sociology and Social Welfare*, 21, 201–219.

Hart, J. (1996). *New Voices in the Nation*. New York: Cornell University Press.

Hattie, J. A., Marsh, H. W., Neill, J. T., and Richards, G. E. (1997). 'Adventure Education and Outward Bound: Out-of-class Experiences That Have a Lasting Effect', *Review of Educational Research*, 67, 43–87.

Henderson, S., Holland, J., McGrellis, S., Sharpe, S., and Thomson, R. (2007). *Inventing Adulthoods. A Biographical Approach to Youth Transitions*. London: Sage Publications.

Holman, T., and McAvoy, L. H. (2005). 'Transferring Benefits of Participating in an Integrated Wilderness Adventure Program to Daily Life', *Journal of Experiential Education*, 27(3), 322–325.

Huebner, A. J. (1998). 'Examining "Empowerment": A How-to Guide for the Youth Development Professional', *Journal of Extension*, 36(6).

Humphrey, R. (1993). Life stories and social careers: Ageing and social life in an ex-mining town, *Sociology*, 27(1), 166–178.

Hur, M. H. (2006). 'Empowerment in Terms of Theoretical Perspectives: Exploring a Typology of the Process and Components Across Disciplines', *Journal of Community Psychology*, 34(5), 523–540.

Jensen, S. Q. (2011). 'Othering, Identity Formation and Agency', *Qualitative Studies*, 2(12), 63–78.

Kohn, S. (1991). 'Specific Programmatic Strategies to Increase Empowerment', *Journal of Experiential Education*, 14(1), 6–12.

Leberman, S., and Martin, A. J. (2004). 'Enhancing Transfer of Learning Through Post-course Reflection', *Journal of Adventure Education and Outdoor Learning*, 4(2), 173–184.

Ledwith, M. (2011). *Community Development: A Critical Approach* (2nd edn). Bristol: Policy Press.

Luckner, J., and Nadler, R. (eds.). (1997). *Processing the Experience: Strategies to Enhance and Generalise Learning*. London: Kendall Hunt.

Mandlebaum, D. G. (1973). 'The Study of Life History: Gandhi', *Current Anthropology*, 14(3), 177–193.

Maynard, L. (2011). '"Suddenly I See" Outdoor Youth Development's Impact on Women's Wellbeing: A Model of Empowerment'. PhD Thesis. Lancaster: Lancaster University.

Mullender, A., Ward, D., and Fleming, J. (2013). *Empowerment in Action: Self-directed Groupwork*. London: Palgrave Macmillan.

Parpart, J. L., Rai, S. M., and Standt, K. (2003). *Rethinking Empowerment: Gender and Development in a Global/Local World*. New York: Routledge.

Prochaska, J. O., and DiClemente, C. C. (1984). *The Transtheoretical Approach: Crossing the Traditional Boundaries of Therapy*. Malabar, FL: Krieger Publishing Co.

Prochaska, J. O., DiClemente, C. C., and Norcross, J. C. (1992). 'In Search of How People Change: Applications to Addictive Behaviours', *American Psychology*, 47, 1102–1114.

Robins, S. P., Chatterjee, P., and Canda, E. R. (1998). *Contemporary Human Behavior Theory: A Critical Perspective for Social Work*. Boston, MA: Allyn and Bacon.

Ryan, R. M., and Deci, E. L. (2000). 'Self-determination Theory and the Facilitation of Intrinsic Motivation, Social Development, and Well-being', *American Psychologist*, 55(1), 68–78.

Sarkin, J. A., Johnson, S. S., Prochaska, J. O., and Prochaska, J. M. (2001). 'Applying the Transtheoretical Model to Regular Moderate Exercise in an Overweight Population: Validation of a Stages of Change Measure', *Preventive Medicine*, 33, 462–469.

Schoon, I., and Bynner, J. (2003). 'Risk and Resilience in the Life Course: Implications for Interventions and Social Policies', *Journal of Youth Studies*, 6(1), 21–31.

Sibthorp, J., and Arthur-Banning, S. (2004), 'Developing Life Effectiveness through Adventure Education: The Roles of Participant Expectations, Perceptions of Empowerment, and Learning'. *Journal of Experiential Education*, 27(1), 32–50.

St Croix, T. (2011). 'Struggles and Silences: Policy, Youth Work, and the National Citizen Service', *Youth and Policy*, 106, 43–59.

Summerson Carr, S. (2003). 'Rethinking Empowerment Theory Using a Feminist Lens: The Importance of Process', *Affilia*, 18(1), 8–20.

Sutton, S. (1996). 'Can "Stages of Change" Provide Guidance in the Treatment of Addictions? A Critical Examination of Prochaska and DiClemente's Model', in Edwards, G. and Dare, C. (eds), *Psychotherapy, Psychological Treatments, and the Addictions*. Cambridge: Cambridge University Press, pp. 189–206.

Taniguchi, S. T., Freeman, P. A., and Richards, A. L. (2005). 'Attributes of Meaningful Learning Experiences in an Outdoor Education Program', *Journal of Adventure Education and Outdoor Learning*, 5(2), 131–144.

Thompson, N. (2007). *Power and Empowerment*. Lyme Regis: Russell House Publishing.

Tyler, I. (2013). *Revolting Subjects: Social Abjection and Resistance in Neoliberal Britain*. London: Zed.

Williamson, H., and Taylor, M. (2005). *Madzinga: Intercultural via Experiential Learning and Outdoor Education. Reflected Experience of a Long-term Training Course in Belgium and Lithuania*. Belgium: Outward Bound.

Zimmerman, M. A. (1990). 'Toward a Theory of Learned Hopefulness: A Structural Model Analysis of Participation and Empowerment', *Journal of Research in Personality*, 24, 71–86.

Zimmerman, M. A. (2000) 'Empowerment Theory: Psychological, Organizational and Community Levels of Analysis'. In Rappaport, J. and Seidman, E. (eds), *Handbook of Community Psychology*. New York: Plenum Press, pp. 43–63.

Part 2

Empowerment and agency: critical examples of practice

Introduction to Part 2: Case studies

This section uses case studies to exemplify the approach developed in the first part of the book. These case studies contextualise our critical framework for practice by bringing to life its key concepts.

The case studies introduce the issue that the programme or project has addressed in its broadest sense, drawing out key injustices to be considered. This will allow you to situate the case study in a wider discourse of social justice and wellbeing. Each case study then details the context, outlining the structures and agency at play. The critical pedagogical approach and process of empowerment within the programmes and projects are then identified.

By understanding the critical pedagogical approach and process of empowerment we can begin to appreciate how the participants in the work developed their awareness of the context, a range of choices of what to do and committed to decisive action(s).

The awareness, choices and actions may be the outcomes of the critical pedagogical work, or may lead to further discernible outcomes. Additional outcomes may comprise changes in the agency of the participants or the structures in which they are situated, and/or changes to wellbeing and social justice.

The analysis of each case is therefore organised by progressing inwards through the concentric circles of the model to ascertain what 'was' before the project or service, and then working outwards through the concentric circles of the model to understand what changes happened as a result of the critical pedagogical work.

The first case study comes from Lucy's Doctoral work at Brathay Trust with young women at risk of sexual exploitation (Maynard, 2011). It was through this participatory action research that the model of empowerment first emerged from practice, which forms the underpinning of the critical framework we present in this book.

The second case study is of a young man from a youth offending programme at Brathay Trust. Lucy took the model to him and he was able to map his experience on to it. This exemplifies how the model was developed and refined in different contexts.

The next two case studies show the application of the model in wider practice beyond where it was developed at Brathay Trust. Firstly, in a school-based charity supporting the engagement of young people by focusing on their well-being needs. Secondly, with the Foyer who support young people who are homeless.

We then broaden the case studies out to include a social action project called the Aspiring Leaders Programme, delivered in partnership between Brathay Trust and the University of Cumbria. Further, we have included a family learning project, which broadens the application of the framework, as well as showing this from a practitioner's perspective.

This leads to the final case study, which is taken from Kaz's Doctoral studies, in which she worked with leaders and managers in a local authority (Stuart, 2013). This participatory action research showed how a newly formed multi-agency team had agency to deal with the structures surrounding them.

References

Maynard, L. (2011). '"Suddenly I See" Outdoor Youth Development's Impact on Women's Wellbeing: A Model of Empowerment'. PhD Thesis. Lancaster: Lancaster University.

Stuart, K. (2013). 'Collaborative Agency Across Professional and Organisational Boundaries in the Children's Workforce in the UK'. PhD Thesis. Lancaster: Lancaster University.

8   A critical pedagogical approach to tackling sexual exploitation

Chapter overview

This case study is based on a programme delivered by Brathay Trust to support young women at risk of sexual exploitation. The chapter describes how and why the young women found themselves in this situation and highlights the importance of awareness of the structures that surrounded the young women as the catalyst for change. The inclusion of a residential within the programme exemplifies how this can be used to step 'away' from everyday contexts to gain a different perspective.

The injustices of sexual exploitation – social justice and wellbeing issues

The Trust for the Study of Adolescence (2000) stated that despite the notion of 'girl power', young women still have lower self-esteem in early adolescence, are unsatisfied with their bodies and find it problematic to say 'no' to sex, or be listened to when saying no. Furthermore, the Mental Health Foundation (2004) found that deliberate self-harm is significantly more common amongst young females than males and there were much higher rates of depression and eating disorders. However, suicide is more common among young males.

Societal pressures penetrate from multiple directions (media, peers, parents) and in multiple ways (appearance, size, clothing and sexuality). This has been found to be an issue across multiple contexts (age, class, economic status and educational attainment). Young women have been seen to lose their 'true' voice (Gilligan, 1993) amongst these conditions in order to fit into the 'right' model of a young woman. This silencing has been seen to have had a significant impact and is damaging to young women's psychological wellbeing.

Some young women's vulnerable wellbeing makes them susceptible to sexual exploitation. Sexual exploitation has likewise been found to affect young women across multiple contexts. A report by the Children's Commissioner for England (2013) found that there were 16,500 children across England in 2011 identified as being at high risk of child sexual exploitation. This gives some sense of the shocking scale of the issue, although the true number of cases is likely to be far higher.

There are some young women who have been found to be more at risk than others, for example young women in the care system. Typically exploiters target young women who may feel more in need of love and attention, because it may have been missing from their lives in care. This is possibly the most common model of exploitation, where this older male will become the young woman's 'boyfriend', supplying love, attention, gifts, alcohol and drugs. They groom the young woman to be dependent upon them, which for the young women may be preferable to the care system they are within. Once dependent, the groomer can more easily exploit the young woman with other men.

However, this is not the only model of exploitation. Aside from the link to trafficking, young women have increasingly been found to be exploited in gangs, by peers and online. In each of these models, young women are groomed and enticed by attention, friendship, parties, drugs and alcohol. Once dependent, because of, for example, finding themselves at a party that they thought would be full of other young people, but is actually full of older men, they may be pressured into staying because of a lack of knowledge of where they are, intoxication and fear.

All of these risks are inter-related: family instability can lead to some young women being placed in the care system, which can make them more susceptible to negative peer influence. Thus young women can have multiple risk factors. These are also directly associated with related situations such as offending, disengagement from education, drug and alcohol misuse, and mental health issues.

The context of this case study: the structures and agency in the situation

The young women were between the ages of 12 and 18, with varying 'risk factors' (defined by their involvement in a local women's service). Commonly they were at risk of being involved, or were currently involved, in being groomed by an exploiter. Their risk of exploitation was equally varied and included having family members involved in sex work or exploitation, being in care, peer influence such as friendships with peers who then pass them on to gangs to be exploited, and through sex for favours (when a young woman will perform a sex act, such as oral sex, in return for somewhere to sleep, a lift home, a cigarette or simply attention). This chapter is based on Lucy's PhD research into how to support young women living in such risky situations.

A significant feature within this programme was the use of residential experiences as time 'away' and a catalyst for change. The residential provided the opportunity for the young women to feel less pressure from society or exploitative relationships and be able to step out and take a meta-view of life. The programme was grounded in outdoor and experiential learning philosophy and practices. Whilst the efficacy of this type of work is well evidenced, it was not without issues. Outdoor youth development can be inaccessible to young women and may typically reflect stereotypical masculine characteristics and assumptions. However, it was exactly this critique that was found to have significant impact. The programme challenged these stereotypes and the young women explored characteristics such as confidence, strength and control, which were in turn linked to agency, social justice and wellbeing.

The critical pedagogical approach and process of empowerment in the programme

There was compelling evidence that the programme's critical pedagogical space and approach enabled empowerment. Getting away was experienced as away from the circumstances the young women were experiencing in their lives, as well as away to a new, exciting and supportive environment. The programme also offered the young women opportunity to develop friendships and positive networks, as one participant said: "... just with everyone supporting me, it felt dead nice, dead good. Everyone was looking out for me and I was safe and everyone was there for me".

The young women showed that they felt good about their achievements, felt trust amongst the group and made realisations about themselves and their lives.

Awareness, choice, action

The young women's stories showed how they were reacting to the world in which they found themselves and appeared out of control of their lives. This was shown in Gemma's story: Gemma was 13 years old and at risk of being exploited as a consequence of her Mum being a sex worker and associated class A drug habit. Gemma rarely attended school, drank alcohol regularly, and ran away from home and her grandparents' care. Gemma cared greatly about her Mum, so much so that sometimes she would pick her up off of the floor when she had used (drugs), laying her on the couch and staying with her in case she overdosed. Gemma was at risk of being exploited by her Mother to have sex with men, to fuel her habit. Gemma's love and loyalty for her Mum was so strong, it made her highly susceptible to this:

> "How can I send me own Mum to jail? Because I still suffer then, because I'm without a Mum! ... I think if I could find a way to change it, I'd change it now. But I can't find a way to change it [laugh]. It seems as if there's no hope, nothing there, nothing to work towards."

Being away represented difference and was a spark for the young women to awaken from a reactive place. Time to reflect, positive experiences of outdoor challenge and the unconditional support of the staff were identified as positive sparks for change.

These sparking moments seemed to bring on realisations for the young women about themselves and their situations. This process involved the young women questioning and challenging the status quo. The staff challenged the young women to ask these questions through the programme of activities. There were realisations that life didn't have to be that way. Another young woman, Bernie, explained:

> *"Coz you know what, I thought, I don't need you [Groomer] anymore. I took a hard look in the mirror at myself and then I looked at him … and I thought, I don't want that. I was like no he's going to love me forever and all this lot. And I just thought I've lost so much, and I thought he never gave me anything back, and I thought [f**k] you I don't need you any more."*

Both Bernie and Gemma's awareness had risen enough for them to realise they wanted to do something about their situations. These were changes that others had been trying to help them achieve, but they had previously fought against. Gemma's Key Worker had tried to work with her to see going into care as positive, but she had fought against it, accepting this was how life was going to be. During the programme Bernie told Gemma about her experiences of living in foster care. It appealed to Gemma that she could see her Mum on her own terms and when her Mum wasn't using. This had been something her Key Worker had suggested, but Gemma had always pushed against.

Upon this realisation and questioning came a sense of wanting. This was a wanting of change, difference or of a more specific goal. It was an intrinsic desire based on a heightened sense of self and situation. This was a wanting of more, better, not to be hurt, a better life, positive attention, someone to love them. Gemma wanted to find out about foster care to change her situation. Three weeks after the programme, Gemma had opened up to the support that social services had previously 'threatened' and was on her way to living with a foster family and going back to school. She said:

> *"I've changed the way I act, my personality, I'm more mature! I know this because of some of the decisions I've had to make, like foster care and leaving my Mum, my Nan, and my family to go and live with someone I don't know."*

This illuminates the power of positive peer networks to spark different possibilities. Bernie also showed how influential the people around her were and the importance of an approach that allowed her to learn for herself rather than being told:

> *"And everyone [back home] was like 'I told you so' and I was like, yeah, but I needed to find out for myself. And I didn't need these people telling me what's right for me and what's wrong and what I should and shouldn't do, because at the end of the day I'm going to find out for myself, I need to find out for myself sort of thing. And learn from me own mistakes."*

In relation to this, Bernie described the combination of getting away, positive networks and an experiential approach, which allowed her to reflect and realise things for herself:

> *"In the middle of nowhere ... all the people there, they don't judge you by like what you wear or what you look like, they judge you by sitting down and getting to know you. And they're just all so kind there ... All the activities we did, not just the outside stuff, but like the workshops and everything, it's just, well it does build your confidence up and I don't think you always realise it, until, well I don't know, but you don't always realise it at first, like with your self-esteem, but like it does help you. And like to make friends along the way as well."*

Wellbeing outcomes

As Bernie alludes to above, the process of awareness, choice, action, in relation to the agency she had in her life, was not only regarding her relationship, but was inter-related to her self-worth. This optimises her developing wellbeing, as she has more awareness of both who she is and what she wants; feeling good and functioning well:

> *"It's like on a chart isn't it? It's like we were at rock bottom first, like I felt like a nobody, and I'm sure other people would put it how they felt about themselves, but like getting on this course, it starts escalating a bit more and more and then it just feels like wow! I mean like this is me, this is who I am, you either like it or you don't. I just can't believe how far we've come. I mean looking back I would of thought I'd never be in a place where I am today, never. At least I thought I would still be hung up on him, and then moved out of county somewhere ... so ... I'd never thought I'd come this far, but we have and looking back I hate that old person, I don't like that old person, no. And this is the new me! I'm more confident, I think more of me self, I'm bubbly ..."*

References

Berelowitz, S., Clifton, J., Firmin, C., Gulyurtlu, S., and Edwards, G. (2013). "If only someone had listened". Office of the Children's Commissioner Inquiry into Child Sexual Exploitation in Gangs and Groups. London: Office of the Children's Commissioner.

Gilligan, C. (1993). *In a Different Voice. Psychological Theory and Women's Development.* London: Harvard University Press.

Mental Health Foundation (2004). Retrieved 1st January 2011, from https://www.mentalhealth.org.uk/a-to-z/s/self-harm.

Trust for the Study of Adolescence (2000). Young People and Gender: A Review of Research. London: Cabinet Office.

9 A critical pedagogical approach to reducing re-offending

Chapter overview

This case study is based on a programme designed to reduce re-offending in a rural local authority. It tells the story of one young man who was living a high-risk life, alcoholic, violent, workless and in trouble with the police. The young man maps his story onto the wellbeing framework, showing how the programme sparked his realisation that life could be different.

The injustices of re-offending – social justice and wellbeing issues.

A new modernity has seen both increased options and increased complexity in life trajectories (Beck, 1992). The transition from youth to adulthood is increasingly non-linear and heterogeneous (Thomson et al., 2002). Margo (2008: 27) states "children find it difficult to cope with the complex adult environment, which is increasing their levels of anxiety and rebelliousness". This can be seen to open the door to the youth justice system, particularly for disadvantaged young people.

Margo (2008) states that whilst socioeconomic factors remain central to explaining why some young people offend, indicators of emotional wellbeing at age 10 (e.g. locus of control, self-esteem, and some behavioural and emotional indicators) have a significant relationship with behavioural outcomes at age 16. This is specifically with regard to anti-social behaviour.

NACRO (2009), however, caution that some commentators have been critical of the 'risk factor paradigm' on the grounds that it focuses on individual deficit as the origin of offending, thereby diverting attention away from structural considerations (i.e. societal factors).

The context of this case study: the structures and agency in the situation

Adam's story exemplifies many of the factors highlighted above. Adam grew up amid chaotic circumstances, including neglect, abuse, alcoholism, drugs and criminal activity. His own words provide the most powerful account of the constraining structures surrounding him:

"Me upbringing; I had a bad-un. I think it was just what I was used to, so as I got older I didn't know different. I knew now't else and then when you start, like I knew I was in the wrong at 13 and stuff, but that was the lifestyle I was in.

Like from a young age, I used to tick school at like five! And my Dad wasn't a very good role model, because you always wanna be like your Dad. But my Dad was in and out of jail, till I was about 11. So from a young age I was taking all that in. Like I'd be in a room with like me Mam, me Dad and all their friends and they were drinking and taking drugs, so that was what I was used to.

I was 12 [when I first got in trouble with the police] I set a bin on fire in the middle of the street. But I can remember as young as six being took home by the police, when I lived with my Mam and Dad, so ... But [Grandad] went awol; give us a couple of slaps. He was strict but I didn't listen to him."

The critical pedagogical approach and process of empowerment in the programme or project

Adam was introduced to the programme through his probation worker. It was voluntary and not part of his order, but he chose to engage. The programme aimed to support 18–25-year-old ex-offenders, or those at risk of offending, towards full-time employment.

The approach was holistic and supportive, with a focus on helping participants develop personal, social and employability skills through participation on a course with a nine-month maximum duration. The course had eight structured community group sessions, a residential at Brathay Trust, and mentoring by a trained volunteer.

Awareness, choice and action

What is particularly interesting about this case study is that Adam was shown the empowerment framework and we jointly mapped his changes onto it. This is how Adam summarised the process:

Realisation:

"You're just going with the flow [reactive]. You have a light bulb moment; what am I doing, I need to change, I'm going nowhere. I thought I'd had enough and was being good for quite a while and then the [programme] came along and I done it and got stuck in and then after that I got locked up! I was doing the programme and then this time last year, [laugh] it was [festival], I had a bit too much to drink and I got locked up, for fighting, but luckily, I didn't get prosecuted or 'owt. So I thought right, I'm gonna have to change. I'm gonna have to use everything I've learnt from the programme and put it into action here and just go for it. I thought I don't

want any more of this. And that turned into another one [light bulb moments] and I thought that's it, final straw."

Wanting:

"The people on the course, I think there was only me that really wanted to change on the course. But the other guys, they were probably in that stage in their life where they didn't want to change. So if they wanted to change the help was there. Just take the help, but they obviously didn't want it and it wasn't the right time for them."

Commitment:

"I think I committed to changing, all together. But growing up as well, that was a big change. I know now I am in control, but there is always this little thing in the back of my head saying I could always go back and do something silly and make a stupid mistake. So that's why I wanted to get away as well. I was just a teenage boy who thought life will sort itself out. But, you have to sort it out yourself. You have to go out and get what you want. So I learnt that. The hard way, but in a good way."

One of the things that supported Adam was the way he was treated. The staff on the programme offered choices, rather than telling him what to do, and they treated him as an equal:

"I think that when you're getting cornered and you're getting attacked and attacked [told what to do] you put a defensive shield up. And I think if ya just talk, like we are now, and given advice and shown; then it's different. So I think it's the way people behave with ya that will influence what you do.

Something I learned from what [youth worker] said: it's not about learning how to do something, it's a feeling that it gives us. He asked us what's the best feeling you've ever had in your life? And I was like, I scored six goals in a football game once and me uncle was watching us, because he's been a big influence in sport. And I scored my sixth goal, and it was a beaut, and I just put my arms in the air and just turned round and shrugged my shoulders as if no one could touch us. And he went, well what you need to do, is you need to take that, fold it up, put it in your top pocket because it's yours and you can use it whenever you want. And he said, just think, why did you feel like that? And I said, I felt like I was on top of the world and like I couldn't do anything wrong and everyone was looking at us like I'd achieved something. And he said, well there you go, that's all you need to think about all the time. And I just thought that's a good way to look at life and I thought I'm gonna use that all the time. Like every day I've achieved something. That's one thing the course taught us was to think positive and give everything a go. And it was like ping, there you go. Just that little conversation was one of the biggest influences on us."

Choice:

"So it's options, but people will only do it if they want to do it. You can advise them, so they've got everything for when they decide to go for it. I'd had a realisation and I wanted to change and I wanted to make the most of the programme. They know what they're doing, so I might as well use what they know to help me."

Transfer:

"Like I was on my last week of probation and I thought probation was keeping me on track and I thought I'm just going to go back to my old ways and I thought NO! No, come on, I can do this. It means I've got no more tags and I can go out and do it for myself. And as I walked through the door she [probation officer] said 'I've got some good news for you. I've got a job application for ya'. And I thought you're winding me up! [laugh] After all that hard work and keeping myself on track and today could be the day. It's like I know I can do it and I just need to get the chance."

Sustain:

"It's the positive attitude, the job, a good lifestyle, a healthy lifestyle. I have a couple of drinks now and again, but I'm entitled. Back then it was every day like carrying on, now maybe once a week a drink. But when I go home, I've prepared for it so, it's alight. So I'm sustaining a lifestyle that I've wanted though for a while."

As a result of the programme and Adam's openness to change, he has become more self-aware, developed support networks, developed healthier habits, gained a job, and learned how to look after himself. These are significant outcomes that have enhanced Adam's wellbeing and equality of opportunity.

Life hasn't been plain sailing. Adam has experienced on-going challenges and at times recycles – drinking and fighting. However, these appear to be shorter lived experiences and he seems to constantly recycle around, engaging in work and training. Interestingly, he mapped frequent cycles in all of which he shows awareness of the influence of alcohol. He states,

"I need to give myself a few kicks up the butt. I'm not as scared to ask for help. I know there's people out there willing to help. Why push them away when they want to help."

References

Beck, U. (1992). *Risk Society: Towards a New Modernity.* London: Sage Publications.
Margo, J. (2008). *Make me a Criminal.* London: IPPR.
NACRO (2009). *Youth Crime Briefing: Some Facts About Children and Young People Who Offend.* London: NACRO.
Thomson, R., Bell, R., Holland, J., Henderson, S., McGrellis, S., and Sharpe, S. (2002). 'Critical Moments: Choice, Chance and Opportunity in Young People's Narratives of Transition', *Sociology*, 36(2), 335–354.

10 A critical pedagogical approach to learning and employability

Chapter overview

This case study is focused on a Youth Specialist Programme, delivered by the Eikon Charity. Eikon are an award-winning charity based in Surrey, UK. Their vision is to develop happy, thriving and resilient young adults who make a positive contribution to society. This case study maps Eikon's Youth Specialist Programme on to the wellbeing framework, exemplifying the ways in which a school-based youth programme supports young people's wellbeing to engage in learning.

The injustices of learning and employability – social justice and wellbeing issues

Young people's experiences of school differ greatly. We feel sure that readers are more than aware of the criticism of the current mainstream school systems that are based on Victorian principles – receiving information whilst kept in order through sitting in rows, timed by bells, and meeting age bound curriculum levels. Not all young people achieve what these systems want to measure them against. Furthermore, there is clear inequity in the UK in the educational attainment of particular groups of young people such as those of low socio-economic status, ethnic minority, with special educational needs, and with English as an Additional Language (ONS, 2016).

Poor educational achievement has been linked reciprocally to a wide range of negative outcomes such as unemployment, poverty and poor health outcomes. It is therefore essential that opportunities to attain are socially just or they will reinforce existing marginalisations and injustices.

The clearest links are drawn between a lack of attainment at school and young people aged 16–24 not in education, employment or training (NEET). A 2016 statistical release showed that there were 865,000 16–24 year-olds – or 12.0% of all young people aged 16–24 – NEET in January–March 2016 in the UK (Delebarre, 2016, 1). This level is above the European average.

Smyth (2011: 4) points out that many schools attribute poor attendance and attainment to 'failing students', where it is perhaps the school that has failed. He goes on to state that, "how we as educators respond to 'willed not learning' (Kohl, 1994: 27) has much to do with how willing we are to challenge educational ..."

It is this injustice in school experience, attainment and employability that Eikon sought to impact. How are all young people supposed to feel good and function well amid these educational injustices? In this sense you cannot divorce educational attainment from wellbeing.

The context of this case study: the structures and agency in the situation

This programme is an example of schools recognising the impact of young people's wellbeing to their educational attainment. The Youth Specialist Programme addresses this by focusing in on understanding young people's lives, in order to understand where their education sits and what is enabling and constraining their learning and attainment. In this sense, it attempts to deal with the structural conditions surrounding the young person, rather than divorce their ability from this. As we have discussed earlier in this book, this approach hopes to help young people have more control of their lives and their learning and education.

Some of the conditions being described by the schools include:

• On-line, mobile and digital safety
• Self-harm
• Vulnerability to child sexual exploitation and developing healthy relationships
• Drug and alcohol/substance abuse
• Risk-taking behaviour
• Bullying
• Underlying family and wellbeing issues

The schools started to question how they can expect young people to learn and attain, if they have these issues going on in their lives? The levels of these needs are exemplified in one school where 17% of the overall student population was known to the designated safeguarding team. Another indicator of potential need was the 36% English as an Additional Language students at another school. Students eligible for Pupil Premium Funding ranged from 7% to 30% across the schools showing that they had a high proportion of disadvantaged students to support. This needed additional resource and a different approach.

The Youth Specialist programme is delivered in partnership with the school. It was seen to complement the school's increasing pastoral role and to help prevent young people's difficulties escalating or falling through a gap in provision. This partnership approach enables the programme to work successfully within the school setting.

Eikon assessed the assets and needs of the young people considered to be vulnerable. The young people stated that they needed support with:

- Family relationships
- Self-esteem
- Friendship issues
- Behaviour
- Emotional health

The critical pedagogical approach and process of empowerment in the programme or project

The Eikon programme is delivered in five schools in Surrey, with a Youth Specialist in each school. It aims to enhance young people's wellbeing and resilience. The outcomes through which the programme achieves this aim are:

- Realisation and awareness of self and situation
- Growing positive sense of self
- Growing positive and supportive relationships
- Improved social and communication skills
- Developing coping strategies

The approach taken to achieve these outcomes was school based, preventative, non-formal and experiential in nature. This was delivered through the following activities:

- One to one support
- Group work
- Support groups
- Trips and residentials
- Youth development board

The activities alone do not bring about change; threaded throughout these activities is the supportive and facilitative approach of the Youth Specialists. The Youth Specialists had a role dedicated to the wellbeing of young people, this contrasted to teachers' roles that focus on the learning needs of the young people. This turns the rhetoric from 'you are failing', to 'what's going on for you and how can we help?'

The Youth Specialists are valued by young people and school staff as:

- Relationship building
- Creating safety and trust
- Listening
- Talking through issues and developing action plans
- Independent of the school

- Sign-posting
- Honest, open and realistic
- Information givers
- Friendly and relaxed
- Consistent
- Non-judgemental
- Confidential

Positioning Youth Specialists within schools ensures that a very large number of young people can easily and privately access support. The working environments are also carefully tailored to convey an informal, relaxed and valuing space, considered 'different' to the rest of the school. Young people state that the welcoming space and having time out is highly important.

Awareness, choice and action

In an evaluation of the programme (Brathay Trust, 2016), young people frequently discuss the ways in which their realisations of self and situation are enhanced through the programme. Some state the importance of realising something for yourself rather than being told it. These realisations were perceived by young people to contribute to them 'growing up' and learning lessons for themselves. This was in relation to a variety of situations, including:

- Anger
- Anxiety
- Risk taking
- Vulnerability
- Negative influences
- Consequences of behaviour
- Aspirations

One young person, who attended the programme over three years ago whilst at school, stated:

> "I was storming out and they told me to go see Eikon, I left there a lot calmer so I could realise maybe walking out of college wasn't going to be my best idea and instead I could work through everything. I think I would have disappeared off [without Eikon] and not made anything of myself ... the problems are still there but I'm dealing with and getting on with my life better which I wouldn't have done before [Eikon]"

Young people frequently state realising they are angry, anxious, risk taking or hanging out in negative peer groups. This is also echoed by the school staff:

"... From what I understand, she has realised she was putting herself at risk .... A lot of the time young people don't realise they are putting themselves at risk ... and I think she's realised she's got more important things to set her mind to, with things like GCSEs coming u p..."

The Youth Specialist's approach facilitates this realisation and helps young people understand why this might be and the impact it might have. They support young people to develop confidence, self-belief and self-esteem. This was often expressed in terms of speaking up for themselves, believing in themselves and engaging in class. They have increased choices, learn new skills and strategies and test out different behaviours, with the ongoing support of the Youth Specialist.

Attendance figures show an overall increase in attendance of 64% from the 2013/2014 to 2014/2015 academic years.

References

Brathay Research Hub (2016). *An Evaluation of Eikon's Youth Specialist Programme.* Ambleside: Brathay Trust.

Delebarre, J. (2016). *Briefing Paper: NEET: Young People Not in Education, Employment or Training.* London: House of Commons Library.

Office for National Statistics (2016). *Which Childhood Factors Predict Low Educational Attainment.* Accessed on 4/8/16 at http://webarchive.nationalarchives.gov.uk/20160105160709/http://www.ons.gov.uk/ons/rel/household-income/intergenerational-transmission-of-poverty-in-the-uk—eu/2014/sty-causes-of-poverty-uk.html

Smyth, J. (2011). *Critical Pedagogy for Social Justice.* New York: Continuum Books.

11 A critical pedagogical approach to homelessness

Chapter overview

This case study is focused on the practice of the Foyer Federation. The Foyer Federation has around 300 housing schemes for young people in housing need across the UK and works with approximately 10,000 young people a year.

The injustices of homelessness – social justice and wellbeing issues

There is limited data shaping our understanding of the causes and scale of homelessness in the UK, or of the outcomes of various interventions (Centre Point, 2015; Homeless Link, 2015). Centre Point mapped the progression of young people through the homelessness system of support in the UK demonstrating a) its complexity and b) the loss of data and lack of understanding of progression routes. Centre Point's own Data Bank (2015: 3) estimates the scale of the youth homelessness in the UK and shows:

- More than 136,000 young people a year in England and Wales present to their local authority asking for help because they are homeless or at risk of homelessness
- At least 30,000 young people experiencing or at risk of homelessness are turned away from their local authority every year in England and Wales

This is a serious issue as homelessness immediately leads to other issues and multiple deprivations. A young person without a home cannot care for themselves appropriately, without an address they cannot gain work or benefits, and without money they are open to a range of risky behaviours. It is therefore essential that homeless young people are supported into a range of accommodation and support as quickly as possible.

The Foyer Federation in the UK works directly in this space. The Foyer Federation is a non-statutory organisation who offer information and guidance, accreditation and assurance to a range of support providers that may work with any of the 30,000 young people living in Foyers across the UK. These provider organisations are working directly with young people who are homeless and offer both housing and personal development to all residents.

The context of this case study – structure and agency

The Foyer Federation is a third sector organisation supporting services that draw funding via their Local Authority from the UK Government's 'Supporting People' grant system. Whilst, over the last decade, this increased funds in the short term, there were unforeseen negative outcomes. Firstly, the Foyers relied less on unrestricted grant funds and became increasingly reliant on the Supporting People grant. This led to a secondary problem as the grant became attached to increasingly tighter conditions. The Foyers had to reach pre-determined targeted populations, often referred by the local authority. Increasingly this included young people feeling 'sent' to live in a Foyer. This meant they were less able to work with young people who were choosing to live in the Foyer on a voluntary basis, often in order to access learning and work and often resulted in a decreasing desire amongst young people to engage in any development offers, as they had felt 'told' what to do.

The Foyer Federation could have continued in this vein, supporting the system, watching their members becoming ever more reliant on centralised funding and tight criteria. However they were dissatisfied with the way their practice had been colonised and felt that it was becoming less effective in enabling young people to develop independently.

Foyers were faced with a choice as to whether to continue drawing down funds, working in a prescriptive way that was not congruent with their values, or to return to their principled practice and leave the funding. This could be high risk in the short term as the Foyers sought alternative sources of funding.

With a great display of organisational agency, the Foyer Federation decided to 'reclaim' its original offer and to encourage and support members to move away from the government grant regime. The reclaimed offer is grounded in principles of critical pedagogy and offers an exciting refreshed way of working for Foyers across the UK from 2016.

The critical pedagogical approach and process of empowerment in the programme

The result is a reclaimed offer that supports the awareness, choices and agency of young people. Significantly, this offer was developed with young people. Groups of residents met and developed a theory of change that documented what was on offer. This displays a critical pedagogical approach to service design, ensuring that the views of young residents are as valid as those of the staff. The rest of this chapter will identify the ways in which the reclaimed offer is also grounded in asset-based thinking and a critical pedagogical approach.

Asset-based work supposes a positive competence-based cycle of working that is person centred. A person identifies that they want to make a change (find housing), they identify the strengths that they have (resilience, resourcefulness), positive expectations are maintained by all stakeholders (this person will succeed), opportunities are provided for development (education, benefits, social skills), these are valued by the young person (that helped, I can now ...) leading to continued development of competencies from enhanced self-belief (I can learn and develop) (McCashen, 2014: 11). This positive asset-based thinking stands in stark contrast to deficit approaches, where people are seen as in trouble, or difficult, because they are homeless. They are categorised by what they lack – poverty, homeless, uncommunicative, anti-social, etc. and are expected to do badly. Issues are the focus of review meetings and opportunities blocked as they are seen as too 'risky' (ibid: 10). It would seem obvious that anyone would thrive more easily in an asset-based programme than a deficit-based one, yet statutory services in the UK do seem to be grounded in a needs-led, targeted, deficit-based approach (Mathie and Cunningham, 2005). Whilst thinking in this way may seem straightforward it can be a challenge to notice how embedded deficit thinking is and to implement asset-based working in practice.

A place that values them

The homes provided for young people need to show they are valued. If young people are thought of as assets then we should house them in accommodation that is in good working and decorative order and where we would live ourselves. Broken, shabby, dirty accommodation says 'you're worth nothing'. Functional, decorative, clean environments, say 'you're worth it'. The Foyer have found that high quality accommodation encourages high quality behaviour.

Welcoming young people

Staff need to openly and warmly welcome young people into Foyers. If they are rushed, stressed, preoccupied or negative, then the young person will probably feel devalued, a problem, or an issue to be gotten rid of. Time and space, and a positive attitude are therefore fundamental from the first contact with the young person onwards. A young person who feels welcomed, seen and valued is way more likely to engage than one who feels like another issue in a busy person's day.

Identifying what led to homelessness

Once the young person is welcomed, it is important to establish how and why they arrived at the Foyer. This conversation is about developing awareness of all the structural forces that led to this point. This conversation is critically important in order to externalise the issue of homelessness, to frame it as something that happened to the young person, rather than something that the young person is as a societal label. This may be a critical step in shifting limiting beliefs and negative self-perceptions.

Identifying assets

From the shared awareness that a range of issues led to the young person experiencing homelessness, then a rich conversation can commence about the skills, knowledge, competencies, peer support and such that enabled the young person to cope and survive in those circumstances. This is the development of a personal asset map.

Setting goals and planning what to do with the young person

The young person is an expert on their own life; they know themselves, what they want and what they can achieve. Practitioners, therefore, cannot plan what they 'should do' and how they 'should' achieve it. The practitioner's role is to facilitate and enable the young person to identify what they want and how they want to get there. The Foyer's theory of change map makes it clear what is on offer at the Foyer that the young person may choose as support.

A 'something for something' deal

The strength of this deal is a critical test of 'Foyerness', as if there is a strong attraction for the young people, they will put a lot in. Practice at the Foyers adopting the reclaimed offer is characterised by this reciprocity, which is starkly different to practice that either rescues or abandons young people. The young person is not given unlimited resources, support or budget. This would be disempowering, rescuing and unrealistic. Rather the young person negotiates what they want to take from the Foyer's offer and what they are prepared to give in return. The young person will 'pay' for their accommodation with their benefits, and will 'exchange' what they take from the offer for commitment, engagement and energy. This makes the commitment stage within the process of empowerment explicit.

Review the progress that the young person has made with the young person

Regular review meetings are grounded in the young person identifying what new assets they can add to their asset map, identifying what they did to achieve them, and what they now know about themselves as a result. This stands in contrast to many organisations measuring the change in a young person that they have made. This approach would commodify the young person and disempower them as the organisation claims attribution for the change that occurred rather than attributing it to the young person.

Working in an asset-based way demands that practitioners are critically pedagogical as it represents such a fundamental shift in the conceptualisation and use of power in a helping relationship. It is also critically pedagogical in approach in that the practitioner is always acting to support the young person's awareness, choices and actions.

References

Centre Point (2015). *Youth Homelessness Data Bank: Beyond Statutory Homelessness*. Accessed on 23. 4. 16 at http://centrepoint.org.uk/media/1690269/0054_yhd_report_full_v12.pdf

Homeless Link (2015). *Young and Homeless 2015*. Accessed on 23. 4. 16 at http://www.homeless.org.uk/sites/default/files/site-attachments/201512%20-%20Young%20and%20Homeless%20-%20Full%20Report.pdf

Mathie, A., and Cunningham, G. (2005). 'Who is Driving Development? Reflections on the Transformative Potential of Asset-based Community Development', *Canadian Journal of Development Studies*, 26(1), 175–186.

McCashen, W. (2014). *The Strengths Approach*. Bendigo, VIC, Australia: St Luke's Innovative Resources.

12 A critical pedagogical approach to social action and leadership

Chapter overview

This case study introduces a leadership development programme called the Aspiring Leaders Programme (ALP). The case study explores the critical pedagogical approach used and the outcomes of the programme.

The injustices of social action – social justice and wellbeing issues

Young people have been criticised for not being politically active and exercising their right to vote. The extent to which political parties are able to engage young people, often appears a secondary discussion. However, in the 2016 Brexit debate, young people were claimed to be a priority part of the campaign – albeit the extent and approach to which is debatable. Although young people were initially criticised for not turning out to vote in Brexit, later statistics revealed the actual number was nearly double early predictions. 64% turned out to vote (Yeung, 2016). Of those 18–24 year olds that did vote, 73% voted to remain in the EU (Kelly, 2016). This was the highest age band voting remain; with remain votes gradually decreasing with age bands. Young people were subsequently found across social media protesting, "Thank you baby boomers for the last nail in my generation's coffin ..." "They've voted for something that's not going to really affect them. They're not going to have to deal with the consequences" (ibid).

Young people were left feeling aggrieved and disillusioned. This illuminates the need to understand how to better engage young people in society. As we have discussed previously in this book, the personal is political and in this sense engaging young people personally in what matters to them is an important first step in engaging them on broader terms, in relation to communities, governance, politics and global affairs.

This realisation underpinned the UK Government's 2015 push on social engagement, action and leadership. They described social action as "people coming together to improve their lives and to solve the problems that are important in their communities" (Cabinet Office, 2015: 2). This includes a wide scope of activity, from informal, simple, everyday neighbourly acts, to formal donations of time and money (ibid: 5). The Government has estimated the value of human capital (skills, knowledge, abilities, social, personality and health attributes) in the UK at £18.4 trillion. As they say: "leveraging just a small part of this could have immense value to public services" (ibid: 10).

This is the language of the Big Society and National Citizenship Service, which have been previously critiqued within this book (see chapter 7). A review of youth social action took place in 2012 (Cleverdon and Jordan, 2015) and since then the National Citizenship Service and organisations such as Step up and Serve have sought to engage young people in social action in the UK. The Government estimates that 40% of young people participate in social action (Ipsos Mori, 2014) and they aim to increase that level to 50% by the year 2020. Young people have therefore been positioned as needing to support and lead social action projects, community life, and stand up and take responsibility for the future society.

There is an obvious important problem within this, as young people have been positioned to stand up and take responsibility for a future society, but this is a society they did not vote for. The extent to which this is socially just, or supports social justice, is debatable.

When young people are asked to create the communities they want for their futures, it brings the role of leadership development into the equation. In relation to the community and voluntary sector, Dame Mary Marsh (2010) stated that a lack of planned and supported development opportunities are hampering the sector's leadership capacity to deal with a rapidly changing environment. There is a growing body of research into the challenges faced by sector leaders in the uncertain and volatile political and economic environment of the developing world (Lewis, 2003; Hailey and James, 2004). Bolton and Gosling (2003) state that workers within the sector tend to be either low paid or voluntary staff and that visionary leadership and inspiration are likely to be important aspects of the role. This literature indicates that there is a case for investment in leadership development within the sector in that there is a lack of leadership skills distinctive to its needs.

The context of this case study: the structures and agency in the situation

The Francis C Scott Charitable Trust (FCSCT) had a vision for a leadership programme to future proof Cumbria and North Lancashire's Voluntary and Charitable Sector (VCS). FCSCT saw the need to make a generational difference in the capability of the region's VCS. This had to make a significant contribution to addressing what had been identified as a low aspiration culture within the region. In partnership with Brathay Trust and the University of Cumbria, the Aspiring Leaders Programme (ALP) was created.

The 2009 Cumbrian Economic Plan found that young people were moving away from the county to seek lifestyle, education, employment and housing opportunities. ALP needed to help redress this by encouraging a number of young people to remain in county with the prospect of becoming leaders of third sector organisations. This needed accreditation to support young people into work-based qualifications, as the county as a whole has a lower proportion of Level 3 and 4 qualifications amongst the working age population, alongside a much higher proportion of basic (Level 1) qualifications than elsewhere in the country.

A study by Warwick University (2002) found that tackling social exclusion and marginalisation amongst young people in Cumbria requires a multifaceted approach. ALP needed to be cognisant of and able to address the complex nature of the social issues that impact on employment aspirations in the county.

Graduates needed to influence, change and challenge their communities and create an entrepreneurial groundswell across Cumbria & North Lancashire. Therefore, personal development and accreditation are important constituent parts of the process for the individuals, and to be sustainable, the approach should be community development based.

ALP sought young adults aged between 18 and 25 who were currently working or volunteering in a VCS organisation in Cumbria or North Lancashire. It invested in those already showing voluntary experience, passion and commitment for community leadership. Valuable progression routes were needed for those often identified in communities as having drive and commitment to create change, but little or no opportunity, or qualifications, to realise their ambitions. ALP aimed to help them become aware of their potential and leadership capabilities. For many this was thought to be beyond their reach.

The critical pedagogical approach and process of empowerment in the programme

The three-year programme leads to a degree in Social Enterprise Leadership. This is a demanding course and many participants, at times, have found themselves at the edge of their capacity. It requires them to juggle work, volunteering, university days, residential weekends, action learning sets, business mentoring, independent study, as well as personal and family life, including parenting. Yet, compared to other university degree cohorts, it has an above average retention rate. This obviously begs the question: how?

There are two clear differentiating factors: firstly, ALP uses a blended approach to learning incorporating elements of experiential, observational and reflective learning. Aspiring leaders must be working or volunteering within the VCS throughout the programme. This blends the continuous application of learning to their context, with bringing their context to the degree programme. This is applied learning involving a process of constantly refining their passion and drive for their community pursuit.

This blended approach asks them to reflect on themselves, in relation to their community. In this sense, it is inextricably linked to the second differentiating factor: wellbeing and personal development are threaded throughout the programme. This is based on Bolden's (2006) centrality of self-awareness and the importance of knowing and leading the self, before leading others. This is mirrored in the structure of ALP, as each year is progressively themed: leading the self; leading the team; leading the community/organisation. Considering the unique conditions described above regarding the requirements of VCS leaders, as well as the demands placed on these students, leadership resilience was a particular theme to the wellbeing thread throughout the programme.

Awareness, choice and action

The participants consistently cited that growth in awareness had the greatest impact on them and in particular was a catalyst in developing resilience. This was described as learning what resilience actually was as a concept; thinking about it more; being more conscious of resilience; and focusing on resilience. This was captured by one participant, who stated,

> *"I look back and realise you don't think about resilience until somebody talks to you about resilience ... You don't realise it until you start to talk about it – it doesn't normally come up in conversation with someone saying 'how resilient are you today'? ... Yeah because life just chucks everything at you and you just deal with it and it's not until somebody actually speaks to you about it or you hear about it. A lot of people might think they are not resilient and never will be but then you talk to them about what it means and they think maybe I am – I think that's what happened to me. Just knowing more about effective resilience and learning more about what it means and then things just slot into place."*

Once the aspiring leaders had become aware of resilience, they started to see it more regularly within a variety of contexts, creating a holistic picture of what it was and meant. Critically, one participant stated that *"I think I am more resilient because I am more aware of it"*.

The participants identified a host of choices and actions they had consciously made in response to their awareness of resilience. These choices and actions were generally described as being proactive rather than passive. For example, one participant described a general shift in thinking, actively looking for things she wants to do and change, rather than having things imposed on her. This personal understanding is clearly the underpinning of social action and leadership.

The participants were selected because of their engagement and commitment to their communities. The programme subsequently asks them to reflect on and question themselves and their communities from within. They are constantly critiquing and refining their leadership within their communities. They are exposed to wider knowledge of different choices for which they can bring to life in their community. For example, they are bringing critical business skills to community leadership, which will support the sector to progress in financially challenging times.

It is these aspiring leaders who will transform our communities and societies of the future. Their increased aspirations have been found to inspire other young people and they are role modelling social engagement. It is these aspiring leaders who will support our communities and the young people within them, to engage and show up to vote for the future they want.

References

Bolden, R. (2006). *Leadership Development in Context Leadership South West Research Report 3*. Available at http://business-school.exeter.ac.uk/research/areas/centres/cls/research/publications/abstract/index.php?id=92 (accessed 20/06/14)

Bolton, G., and Gosling, N. (2003). *Passionate Leadership – The Characteristics of Outstanding Leaders in the Voluntary Sector – What Sector Leaders Think*. London: ACEVO.

Cabinet Office (2015). *Harnessing the Potential*. London: Cabinet Office.

Cleverdon, J., and Jordan, A. (2015). 'In the Service of Others: A Vision for Youth Social Action for 2020'. Accessed on 22/4/17 at: https://www.gov.uk/government/publications/a-vision-for-youth-social-action-by-2020

Hailey, J., and James, R. (2004). 'Trees Die from the Top, International Perspectives on NGO Leadership Development', *Voluntas: International Journal of Voluntary and Nonprofit Organisations*, 15(4), 343–353.

Ipsos Mori on behalf of Cabinet Office (2014). *Youth Social Action in the UK – 2014*. London: Cabinet Office.

Kelly, J. (2016). 'Brexit: How much of a generation gap is there?', BBC News Magazine, 24 June, 2016. Accessed at: http://www.bbc.co.uk/news/magazine-36619342

Lewis, D. (2003). 'Theorising the Organisation and Management of Non-govermental Development Organisations. Towards a Composite Approach', *Public Management Review*, 5(1), 325–344.

Marsh, M. (2010). 'Skills and Leadership in the VCSE Sector: Dame Mary Marsh Review'. Accessed on 23/4/17 at: https://www.gov.uk/government/publications/skills-and-leadership-in-the-vcse-sector-dame-mary-marsh-review

Warwick University (2002). 'Youth Labour Market in Cumbria', *Institute for Employment Research Bulletin No. 65*. Warwick: Warwick University.

Yeung, P. (2016). 'EU referendum: Turnout among young voters "almost double" initial reports', *Independent*, 10 July, 2016. Accessed at: http://www.independent.co.uk/news/uk/politics/eu-referendum-brexit-turnout-young-voters-youth-vote-double-a7129181.html

13 A critical pedagogical approach to family work

Chapter overview

This case study describes the challenges of a practitioner finding a critical peda-gogic approach to working with families amid an unjust and damning political agenda, where little structural change was possible. The chapter makes the point that an authentic approach to teaching and learning, involving awareness, choice and action, has efficacy even in situations with multiple contexts and barriers to agency. It acknowledges the need for practitioners to operate authentically even when this appears incongruent with dominant forms of 'best practice'.

The injustices in families – social justice and wellbeing issues

Families have often been under media and government scrutiny and the focus of remedial policy measures in the UK. Common claims are that parents have low levels of skills (HM Treasury, 2006), poor parenting (Phillips, 2013), and social "problems" (Bingham, 2013).

The Leitch Review (HM Treasury, 2006: 39) found that 7 million adults lack functional numeracy and 5 million lack functional literacy. The report links the acquisition of basic skills to employability and GDP. This creates a national economic drive for parents to gain basic skills and the commodifi-cation of human beings into human resources, stating, "Social deprivation, poverty and inequality will diminish" (ibid: 4). The discussion of global wellbeing earlier in this book disputes the claim that more money equates to less inequality. One of the results of this report has been funded family edu-cation in every local authority in the UK, aimed at improving the literacy and numeracy skills of adults and driving employability.

As well as a focus on basic skills, parenting was also critiqued as leading to youth violence (Richardson, 2012), poor educational attainment (Paton, 2013) and the breakdown of society (Bingham, 2013).

These reports spotlight the 'problems' with parents and shift responsibility from the state to an amorphous group of people: 'bad parents' with sensa-tionalist stories (Phillips, 2013). The discourse encourages othering and social abjection (see chapter 5).

The Troubled Families policy is a clear example of the manifestation of these societal views of parents. Then Prime Minister, David Cameron, aimed to "turn around" 120,000 "troubled families" in the UK (DCLG, 2011: 1). The financial driver for this policy was evident from the outset with these families cited as costing the public purse £9 million a year (ibid). To reinforce this message, local authorities who could evidence positive outcomes would be "paid by results" under a complex financial framework. The ills that they were tackling, and payable outcomes included households who:

- Are involved in crime and anti-social behaviour
- Have children not in school
- Have an adult on out of work benefits
- Cause high costs to the public purse (ibid: 2).

Although with every local authority tackling this agenda investment in families grew, the policy further labels and stigmatises families as "troubled". Further, the outcomes above did not account for the underpinning complexities and difficulties. It is not surprising that an independent evaluation of the programme found "no discernible impact on the percentage of adults claiming out-of-work benefits" and "no obvious impact on the likelihood that adults were employed" 12 or 18 months after starting on the programme (O'Carroll, 2016). This focus takes away from the good work that had been achieved to support families, which goes unmeasured and unnoticed. In particular it does not allow us to learn best practices, innovation, or the proximal outcomes that are the stepping stones to these more distal and societal outcomes.

In many respects practitioners are the interface between these discourses of 'bad' parents and 'troubled families' encoded in policy and programmes, and the parents labelled as such.

The context of this case study – structure and agency

Family learning in the UK is often focused on the acquisition of English, maths and language skills by the whole family (FEML). This case study documents Charlotte's practice delivering FEML programmes in a range of primary schools in North West England. The schools identify and invite parents to take part in a 10-week FEML course focused on one of the core subjects. The programmes are funded by the Skills Funding Agency whose aim is to increase the employability of parents by enhancing their basic skills. FEML is therefore discretely political, as it addresses the needs of the employment market by 'upskilling' adults.

This functional or utilitarian approach to learning sits in opposition to emancipatory ideals of education as liberatory and self-directed. Whilst the agenda of the funder constrains the curriculum of the programme, it enables the provision to happen, which may be beyond the resources of the school otherwise. The school uses the funding to provide a family oriented programme with an agenda of enhancing pupil attainment by increasing parents' basic skills, meeting the demands of its inspection body, Ofsted.

Typically, the funding agency's requirements for providers to meet "community learning measures" focus on the number of qualifications achieved in functional skills exams. Ravitch (2011) suggests that this may be distorting the educational process, narrowing the curriculum, and conflicting with the goals of meaningful education. Such a narrowing of the curriculum can lead to use of abstract and inauthentic materials that families struggle to see the point of.

These agendas may or may not align with the hopes and expectations of the parents enrolling on the FEML course. There is a wide range of parental motivations and attitudes, some are active participants in school, some are passive customers, whilst others may be avoidant.

It was Charlotte's dissatisfaction with this narrow, decontextualised and abstract learning that led her to focus on a different way of practising – authentic learning. This meant using meaningful tasks that had relevance to the families' lives. Charlotte was inspired by Freire's proposal of emancipatory education (Freire, 1974) and Habermas's (1987) ideas of 'lifeworlds'. This challenges how taken for granted assumptions about who we are, can be used to inform meaningful and personal choices about learning.

With this realisation, Charlotte chose to apply authentic concepts to her family learning practice and used her individual agency to develop a critically pedagogical way of delivering FEML – authentic family learning.

The critical pedagogical approach and process of empowerment in the programme

Charlotte identified six key practices that enabled her to overcome the systemic oppression of parents and practice from central government agendas.

Who we are – authentic lifeworlds

In the FEML environment there are generally four participants: practitioner, primary school teacher/staff, parent and child. Each has different lifeworlds, which the authentic practitioner identifies and understands in order to support their interaction. The lifeworlds are the shared values that evolve over time in a range of social groups. This encompasses a range of suppositions about who we are and what we value about ourselves, what we believe, what shocks and offends us, what we aspire to, what we desire and what we are willing to sacrifice (UC Calgary, n.d.).

In authentic family learning none of these lifeworlds is privileged above another, although power is disproportionately allocated and therefore always relevant. The authentic practitioner has to convey equal value to all and tackle difficulties up front.

Third space – authentic place

Adults can have negative experiences of classrooms and therefore entering a primary school, with its gates, intercom and bells, can be daunting and can trigger an evocative set of sometimes painful memories.

Given that this is where FEML takes place, the authentic practitioner has to acknowledge this and create a different space. This includes adult size furniture and equipment, perhaps arranged in a circle or U-shape, rather than rows.

Family learning spaces include parents and children as partners in their learning. This is a productive, focused and busy space, where parent and child actively work together to achieve a shared and meaningful goal.

Shared goal – authentic agendas

It is fundamental to establish shared goals and focus on real tasks. This may be very different to previous deficit approaches and may therefore be a challenge, or a delight, for families to experience truly shared goal setting.

The authentic practitioner establishes trust and builds constructive relationships with families in order to agree a shared goal that works for everyone. This is facilitated by a slowing down of 'the business' of establishing a course and investing time in rapport building and the emerging agendas. This is purposeful time invested in unearthing the parents', rather than schools', interests.

The practitioner seeks to retain professionalism but shed hierarchy. The use of first names, signifying equity and difference to normal primary school practice, is significant, as well as establishing shared leadership where the practitioner becomes part of the group.

Meaningful activities – authentic actions

The authentic practitioner is deeply curious about the lives of the families in order to plan what 'meaningful' activities might look like. The materials and tasks need to be authentic, for example, searching online about a local change that would impact on the family, looking for a job, or researching a trip together.

The ranges of discrete literacy tasks within these shared activities were all real. This task included the parents' interests, a wide range of real choices and the parents carrying out the actions. Alongside the gains in literacy, it is questioning why they are in these situations, or why these tasks are meaningful to them. This enables families to develop critical consciousness.

Intent on real relationships – authentic relating

Family learning is special because of the relationship between child and parent. This bond provides a sense of legitimacy to parent learners, giving them the 'right' to be in the class. Those who lack confidence in their parenting or literacy skills, have the legitimising moment where the child comes running in, looking for and claiming their parent.

This is built on through shared goals and authentic learning. Activities, such as fundraising for the school, can give the family learning group a special status in the school as they work towards their shared goal in a public manner. Again this legitimises children leaving class to go to family learning group. It has special status that has a bolstering effect on the relationships between participants who share in this distinct experience.

The rejection of inauthentic and deficit learning by, for example, avoiding the use of initial assessment that emphasises the adults' lack of skills rather than uncovering their abilities, can sometimes create a vacuum, where previously conflict might have existed. The lack of hierarchy and imposed activity can also create suspicion and confusion as the accepted role of teacher and student are not being taken up. This is challenging for the practitioner, who should maintain a focus on authenticity, shared goals, the enjoyment and engagement with the children.

Radical practice – authentic reflection

This pursuit of critical consciousness, in which power structures are revealed, has radical potential in that parents and children are invited to acknowledge and critique structures and reflect on the impact of these on their agency. This may involve questioning the legitimacy of authority figures. Mindful and focused facilitation of these types of discussions is essential to avoid devolving into a generalised and circular airing of grievances.

It is essential that the practitioner maintains a neutral role across all interactions in the school, so as to be accepted as a peer by staff. This can occur in parallel to them being accepted as an ally of the parents, who they see as distinct from, but able to communicate with, school staff as a useful advocate for perceived injustices. Therefore, reflective practice is essential to the authenticity of the practitioner to all parties.

Wellbeing outcomes

Through this type of practice Charlotte observed a number of wellbeing outcomes over time. They fall loosely into two domains: effecting personal change and effecting wider societal change.

Learners felt change personally, gaining confidence, communication, collaboration and leadership skills. This feeling of self-worth fuelled their functioning, for themselves, their families, and wider society. For example, in one setting learners identified a desire to develop more accuracy in their writing as they were creating publicly displayed posters and flyers. This showed a confidence in not only asking for help, but to have their work made public. The confidence of the learners increased so much that they wrote to their local MP and, with some glee, proofread and edited his response. Their new-found skills and agency had enabled them to start expressing their views in order to influence social change.

References

Bingham, J. (2013). 'Blame bad parents for Britain's ills says Sir Michael Wilshaw', *The Telegraph*, accessed on 24. 9. 16 at: http://www.telegraph.co.uk/news/uknews/10381632/Blame-bad-parents-for-Britains-ills-says-Sir-Michael-Wilshaw.html

DCLG (2011). *The Troubled Families Programme*. London: DCLG.

Freire, P. (1974). *Education for Critical Consciousness*. London: Continuum.

Habermas, J. (1987). *Theory of Communicative Action, Volume Two: Lifeworld and System: A Critique of Functionalist Reason*. Translated by Thomas A. McCarthy. Boston, MA: Beacon Press.

HM Treasury (2006). *Leitch Review of Skills*. London: HMSO.

O'Carroll, L. (2016). '£1.3bn troubled families scheme has had "no discernible impact"', *The Guardian*, accessed on 24. 9. 16 at: https://www.theguardian.com/society/2016/aug/08/13bn-troubled-families-scheme-has-had-no-discernible-impact

Paton, G. (2013). 'Poor parenting "linked to underachievement in schools"', *Telegraph Education News*, accessed on 24. 9. 16 at: http://www.telegraph.co.uk/education/educationnews/9837864/Poor-parenting-linked-to-underachievement-at-school.html

Phillips, A. (2013). 'Worst mum in the UK and the plague of bad parenting', *The Mirror*, accessed on 24. 9. 16 at http://www.mirror.co.uk/news/uk-news/worst-mum-britain-plague-bad-1835987

Ravitch, D. (2011). 'If You Believe in Miracles', Education Week's Blog: Bridging Differences, Accessed on 24. 9. 16 at: http://blogs.edweek.org/edweek/Bridging-Differences/2011/10/if_you_believe_in_miracles_don.html

Richardson, H. (2012). 'Poor Parenting "fuels rise in violent behaviour"', BBC News, accessed on 24. 9. 16 at: http://www.bbc.co.uk/news/education-17553210

UC Calgary (n.d) '*Notes on Habermas: Lifeworld and System*'. Available at: http://people.ucalgary.ca/~frank/habermas.html Accessed on: 05. 10. 16

14 A critical pedagogical approach to practitioner development

Chapter overview

This case study draws from Kaz's Doctoral studies which used participatory action research (PAR) to explore the leadership activity of leaders and managers in the children's workforce in a local authority. This critical pedagogical approach unearthed that leaders and managers with high levels of critical consciousness have more agency. It illuminates the role of reflection within this approach in levering that critical consciousness.

The injustices of practice – social justice and wellbeing issues

Children's Services in the UK have responsibility for the wellbeing of children, young people and families. They have particular accountability for those who are vulnerable and at risk. In the 2000s, a series of deaths of children through neglect and abuse triggered a review of the way in which services worked.

There was a national perception that Children's Services were not looking after the wellbeing of children and that this was unjust. Public and political outcry led to a restructuring of services.

The Children's Act 2004 and the Every Child Matters policy mandated that professionals from education, health and social care should work together in order to better protect children and young people. This was as a direct result of poor information sharing playing a part in the children's deaths. Integrated working was introduced across the UK predominantly as a structural arrangement.

The context of this case study – structure and agency

This integrated working agenda is the context for this critical pedagogical work. The new working structure was imposed on practitioners from different disciplines. Many of them were challenged, bewildered and uncertain of how to do this in a short space of time, without any release from the everyday demands of their jobs, with colleagues that they had never worked with before.

This case study describes an example of 10 leaders making sense of this policy change throughout a yearlong PAR project. The leaders were from education, health, social care, policing, family services and further education. They came together on four occasions to jointly plan workforce development across the newly amalgamated 'children's workforce' in a local authority.

The critical pedagogical approach and process of empowerment

The roots of PAR are entwined with critical pedagogy. Of fundamental significance is that the research process is 'with' rather than 'on' people (Denscombe, 2001). Kemmis and McTaggart (2005) outline three components used to define PAR:

1   Shared ownership of research projects
2   Community-based analysis of social problems
3   An orientation toward community action.

The leaders were all responsible for the services that they were designing, yet they were working together as a community of practice that all wanted positive outcomes for children, young people and families. The four sessions involved the leaders sharing and reflecting on their experiences, conceptualising it, and analysing and interpreting it. In this respect they participated in the full range of research activities.

Kaz facilitated the PAR sessions. In PAR the researcher is involved in rich dialogue rather than remaining independent and detached; "the researcher becomes a listener who encourages the dialogue to continue" (Harper, 1998 in Gauntlett, 2007: 35). This is congruent with Freire's (1970) co-intentional learning. Working with the participants "articulate[d] democratic norms and values; the importance of everyone having a voice, being listened to carefully, and heard with respect" (Gilligan, 2011: 24). Sharing experiences at times challenged the leaders' individual assumptions of 'reality' and at other times supported them, validating that they were not alone – the foundation of collective action.

Use of creative research tools enabled this co-construction of meaning between the leaders. Such tools are well theorised within action research (McNiff *et al.*, 1996; McIntosh, 2010; Brinton Lykes, 2001; Mienczakowski and Morgan, 2001; Martin, 2001; Gauntlett, 2007: 70). Creative tools can elicit depth of meaning because they stimulate double reflection in the recall, interpretation and reconstruction of events (Moon, 2004).

Awareness, choices and action

The group engaged with personal and group tasks about collaboration. The tasks enabled the leaders to develop a shared awareness of the context. Individual reflective activities stimulated dialogue about shared conceptual terms of reference. For example, they created three-dimensional physical maps of the membership of the new integrated working team. Drawing a boundary on a sheet of A3 paper, they selected random objects to represent each member of the team and 'placed' them inside the boundary, wherever they felt they should be. This technique is called 'imago mapping' and has roots in transactional analysis. Eric Berne (1963: 223–232) first used the concept to make the private psychodynamic structure of groups and teams visible.

The participants engaged in this task in a playful way and there was laughter and wry smiles as they created their maps. Rich dialogue was used to explore what the maps might signify, revealing marginalisation and oppression between team members. The maps enabled the leaders to discuss the team that they were in from a distance. Their comments were not about individuals, but about 'it' – the team. The three-dimensional activity revealed much about the nature of the dynamics within the team and reinforced trust and openness as team members accepted one another's comments without hostility or defensiveness.

Further sessions included an activity theory mapping workshop (Engeström, 2001). Activity theory maps make clear what is taking place, who is doing it, and what is controlling it. From these analyses it became clear to what extent the 'system' of people and tasks mutually support the intended outcome, or the contradictions that get in the way. The activity theory map below shows how the activities of two organisations is hopefully complementary, contributing to outcomes together.

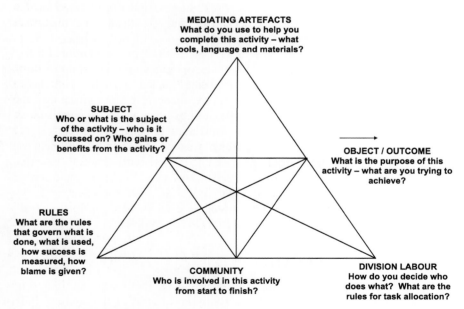

Figure 14.1 Third generation activity theory diagram (developed from Engeström, 2001:136).

Kaz facilitated the leaders' analysis with a set of tailored questions. The leaders recorded their reflections on an individual activity theory map representing their organisational perspective. Dialogue on the individual maps revealed that many of them contained contradictions, blockages and confusion within each organisation and particularly between organisations. Not only did this lead to insights and awareness, it also led into discussion of what needed to change and what could be different to enhance outcomes. This showed the leaders moving from enhanced awareness of structures, to emerging awareness of choices that they could make individually and jointly.

Through participating in the sessions the leaders identified a range of factors that enabled them to achieve their intended outcomes (integrated working) and those that constrained them. From this knowledge the individuals and team as a whole were able to develop strategies to overcome or limit the constraining factors, and capitalise and lever the enabling factors.

In other words, the awareness that they developed of their situation enabled them to make clearer choices and led to them taking decisive actions. The sessions had been empowering and had enhanced their agency. This sense of collective agency enabled the leaders to work more effectively together.

Wellbeing outcomes

As a result of participating in the research it was clear that the leaders felt better about themselves and their abilities. They had increased the professional trust within the group, shared diverse perspectives and validated one another's feelings of isolation, frustration and fear. As such, their professional wellbeing had arguably increased.

In addition the team of leaders developed a workforce development strategy for the Local Authority. This included developmental activities that would enable different agencies to understand one another and to develop integrated working processes from the front line. The impact of the workforce development strategy is not known, but it is hoped that this will have enhanced the ability of staff to work together which will in turn have enhanced outcomes for children, young people and families. As such, this small piece of critical pedagogy with professionals can be seen to support social justice.

References

Berne, E. (1963). *The Structure and Dynamics of Organisations and Groups.* New York: Ballantine Books.

Brinton Lykes, M. (2001). 'Creative Arts and Photography in Participatory Action Research in Guatemala', in Reason, P. and Bradbury, H. (eds) *Action Research: Participatory Enquiry and Practice.* Sage: London, pp. 363–371.

Denscombe, M. (2001). *The Good Research Guide. For Small-scale Research Projects.* 2nd edn. Maidenhead: Open University Press.

Department for Education (2004). *The Children Act.* London: HMSO.

Engeström, Y. (2001). 'Expansive Learning at Work: Toward an Activity Theoretical Reconceptualization', *Journal of Education and Work*, 14(1), 133–156.

Freire, P. (1970). *Pedagogy of the Oppressed*. London: Penguin.

Gauntlett, D. (2007). *Creative Explorations*. London: Routledge.

Gilligan, C. (2011). *Joining the Resistance*. Cambridge: Polity Press.

Kemmis, S., and McTaggart, R. (2005). "Participatory Action Research: Communicative Action and the Human Sphere', in Denzin, N. K. and Lincoln, Y. S. (eds) *The Sage Handbook of Qualitative Methods* (3rd edn.). London: Sage, pp. 559–604.

Martin, A. (2001). 'Large Group Processes as Action Research', in Reason, P. and Bradbury, H. (eds) *Action Research: Participatory Enquiry and Practice*. London: Sage, pp. 200–208.

McIntosh, P. (2010). *Action Research and Reflective Practice: Creative and Visual Methods to Facilitate Reflection and Learning*. London: Routledge.

McNiff, J., Lomax, P., and Whitehead, J. (1996). *You and Your Action Research Project*. London: Routledge.

Mienczakowski, J., and Morgan, S. (2001). 'Ethnodrama: Constructing Participatory, Experiential and Compelling Action Research through Performance', in Reason, P. and Bradbury, H. (eds) *Action Research: Participatory Enquiry and Practice*. London: Sage, pp. 219–227.

Moon, J. (2004). *A Handbook of Reflective and Experiential Learning*. Oxon: Routledge Falmer.

15 Critical pedagogical practices

Chapter overview

Throughout this book we have given examples of critical pedagogical approaches in practice. This chapter will describe some of these examples in more detail. Each section provides an overview of where the practice came from and a short description of what it might look like. Further reading is given as a key resource signposting to other more extensive ideas and toolkits.

Third spaces

The term 'third space' is used to refer to the spaces where two cultures may come together in a neutral zone, originating from descriptions of the space created between indigenous and colonial people in countries across the world (Saleha Gandana, 2008). Later studies focused on how a third space between the home and the workplace could be a useful space for learning, free from the formal constraints of work/school, and also free from the informal constraints of home or community (Pahl and Kelly, 2005).

Gutierrez (2008) examined the third spaces needed to enable migrants in the USA to learn. He discovered that they could not just 'slot into' Western society or learning institutions, and so created a space that accounted for all their different experiences and approaches to learning and that allowed them to explore and develop their identities. In this space, Gutierrez found "students begin to reconcile who they are and what they might be able to accomplish academically and beyond" (ibid: 148).

The third spaces that Gutierrez created were not just geographically neutral; they were also as free as possible from the assumptions of other cultural spaces. They featured dialogue, debate, story-telling, metaphor, art and theatre work in order for the participants to create their own cultural norms.

Learning in these contexts can be transformative as they enable participants to challenge the taken for granted practices of everyday life (ibid: 151). Questioning what is taken for granted and how these norms are controlled in daily dialogue leads to understanding of power (Moje *et al.*, 2004). Importantly, these can represent 'safe spaces' free from judgement and oppression where self-expression and exploration is valued (Hill Collins, 1990).

What does this theory offer the critical pedagogue? It suggests that the environment in which sessions take place is as important as the activity in the session itself. The group need to work in a space that is as free from the hegemonic controls of society as possible. One dimension is physical space or geography, thus a session may need to be distant from or between home, work, school, church and other places of influence. A second dimension may include the physical artefacts in the space. Ideally the building, furniture, posters, décor would not reinforce any layers of power or remind the group of places of influence. The layout of the furniture is important, as the positioning of chairs or even a variety of chairs can be used to convey power.

Facilitators need to consider carefully how they use the space to remain with the group rather than sitting or standing above or in front of the group. The routines and rituals employed in the space are also important, creating a space that equally values and respects everyone – regardless of the range of differences encompassed within the group.

For us, the term 'third space' equates to a 'neutral space' which is as free of hegemony as possible in terms of place, structure, appearance, positioning and rituals. Although hard to achieve, it is essential to consider.

Dialogue

Why do we use the word 'dialogue' rather than talking, or conversation? What special additional meanings come from this word? The word has several meanings, the one that we draw on implies that there is an exchange of ideas and that both parties are willing to listen to one another fully and respond to one another fully. This is not a cosy 'chat', it's not gossip, banter, nor is it point scoring or an argument. It is a very specific form of conversation.

The word originated from the Greek language where the phrase διά or dia means through and λόγος or logos means speech and reason. Dialogue therefore means learning through speech and reasoning. The first extensive use of the term was by Plato who wrote dialogues featuring the character Socrates. This is where the phrase 'socratic dialogue' comes from. These dialogues would tackle moral or philosophical issues.

Freire (1970) emphasised that critical pedagogical learning was grounded in dialogue. He states, "without dialogue there is no communication and without communication there can be no true education" (Freire, 1973: 65). This dialogue was a discussion with people, rather than an educator telling people what they should learn. This dialogical learning is full of problem posing that Freire asserts leads to conscientisation, the increasing self-awareness and political awareness of those in dialogue. Dialogical learning is egalitarian with the views of all participants valued, perceptions exchanged and new meanings developed.

The key characteristics of dialogue include:

1   Knowledge isn't fixed – it means different things to different people in different times and places
2   The exchange of different perspectives leads to new understandings and new knowledge
3   Learners are fully engaged in environments where these differences are respected and rigorously explored
4   Meanings are constructed from the inside by learners in dialogue, rather than imposed from the outside, creating powerful learning
5   Learners gain content knowledge and improved thinking skills
6   Learners respect one another
7   Personal experiences and ideas are both validated and challenged
8   The exertion of power is explored along with scope for personal and collective action
9   New meaning emerges from the shared perspectives

(adapted from educNET, 2016).

This list shows how dialogue is much more than talking. This brings us to the first key point – it is a skill that needs to be learnt. It is not a high level skill, it is not reliant on intelligence, but it is reliant on self-control, reflection and thinking skills. The participants have to be still enough and present enough to be able to listen. They need to process what they have heard and not pass judgement on it. They need to reflect on what it might mean and offer ideas, thoughts, questions and personal experiences back. The themes that emerge from the dialogue were traditionally called 'generative'. As Ledwith (2016: 53) says, they are "'generative' as they generate passion because they are relevant to people's experiences, and that releases energy from the apathy of hopelessness that comes from having no control over life's circumstances".

Initial attempts at dialogue might therefore be short and sharp, or you might break down and explain each of the different components and teach young people how to listen and how to express themselves. Ryan (2016) summarises seven skills needed to engage in dialogue:

1   Deep listening
2   Respecting others
3   Inquiry
4   Voicing ideas openly
5   Suspending assumptions and judgements
6   Balancing voicing and inquiry
7   Reflecting.

These may need to be 'taught' before the group can engage in the non-taught dialogue! Over time their ability to engage in and sustain dialogue will increase. It is worth stressing that the experience of dialogue is more important than the quality of the dialogue, and quality will follow quantity.

It may also be surprising for CYPF to be engaged in a dialogue – they may be very used to being lectured and told what to do, they may be used to getting the upper hand with wit and banter, or volume and pace of speech, they may be used to being quiet and not taking part. All of these forms of communication are laden with power. Someone gains the upper hand, wins the floor, and has the last word. True dialogue has none of these dynamics, no games, no winners and losers, and this can be disconcerting.

Dialogue is often supported by the existence of a safe space, a third space. This links these two key concepts together. Feeling safe promotes the ability to engage in dialogue as trust amongst a group is built. The groups of people who engage in dialogue in a critically pedagogical way were traditionally called 'culture circles' (Souto-Manning, 2009; Freire, 1973).

What does this theory offer the critical pedagogue? Whilst it is simple enough to understand that dialogue is an egalitarian exchange of ideas, it may be hard to put into practice. Careful explanation, development of sub-skills, experience and ground rules may be needed initially. Dialogue is the prime tool of critical pedagogy and so it is worth investing the time in understanding how to develop and promote this form of learning.

Narratives

Rather like the section above, you might wonder what the difference is between a narrative and a story.

A story is a direct telling of events, in sequence as they happen. A narrative, on the other hand, is a re-telling of a story. The events may be put in a different order, altered, and certain things emphasised or portrayed in a particular way. A narrative is therefore not necessarily true to events. Most of the 'stories' that we tell are probably narratives, for example after an altercation at work I may well alter events for a dramatic retelling when I get home – this is natural and does not make the story any less valid. In terms of meaning, the narrative elements add additional meaning; they show what happened and how important those events were to me by what is kept, removed or edited in the narrative process. Although we all tell narratives, the word is rather cumbersome, and so 'stories' is used in everyday speech.

Humans have told stories for millennia, and indeed used them to pass on the heritage of their own cultures (Chisholm, 2000). As individuals we experience stories from childhood; for many people, they act as one of our earliest forms of education, encouraging us to develop an ethical sense and to see relations between our lives and the wisdom of others. Even if we are not told stories at home, we are exposed to them in school, among peers and colleagues, and through popular culture (for instance, television, computer and music). They are an intrinsic part of being human. Stories are not just a pastime, but also a developmental tool. As Clandinin and Connelly (1994: 415) state:

> Stories are the closest we can come to experience as we and others tell our experience. A story has a sense of being full, a sense of coming out of a personal and social history .... Experience ... is the stories people live. People live stories and in the telling of them reaffirm them, modify them, and create new ones

A good story moves us, teaches us, and transforms us (Campbell, 1968; Chisholm, 2000; Kouzes and Posner, 2003). By providing metaphors to challenge behaviour, Vogler (2007) maintains that stories become almost alive for listeners, who participate in the creation of a dramatic experience. The inherent power of stories is well known within child development and educational research (Bettelheim, 1976). Stories are also used as a tool for adult learning (Parkin, 2001), organisational development (Denning, 2005) and even as a discrete mode of research (Clandinin and Connelly, 2000). Narrative is particularly useful across all these contexts to access affective dimensions of experience (Thomas and Killick, 2007).

'Narrative therapy' is a widely used therapeutic tool to support development through 're-authoring' or 're-storying' (Morgan, 2000: 12; White, 2007). Like other therapeutic approaches, narrative therapy seeks to be a respectful, non-blaming approach which centres people as the experts in their own lives. It views problems as separate from people and assumes people have many skills, competencies, beliefs, values, commitments and abilities that will assist them to reduce the influence of problems in their lives. As Walther and Carey (2009: 2–3) point out, narrative therapy supports people to develop a 'concept of their life' that will build an intentional identity, sense of direction and agency. These, they state, are important to enable 'becoming' and interacting with structure rather than just 'being' in structures.

Ledwith (2005) identifies the importance of personal narratives as a process by which the personal can become political. Ledwith describes her interest in ordinary, everyday, small stories. These are situated against the grand narratives or discourses that tell people how to live their lives. When shared, the small stories show personal oppressions or sites of struggle within the grand narratives that surround us and the oppressions that thwart us.

Shared, these stories validate, they enable internalised problems to become appropriately externalised, and they create support networks. What was an individual's story of failure turns into a shared story of oppression. The collective narrative changes the way that the world is viewed. This may well be enough, however, seeing the world in a different way may lead to a new way of being and acting in the world – and this can then bring about social change. For Ledwith (2005) this is collective action for social justice. Story telling can support collective action in the following ways:

- Sharing and listening – people need confidence to share their stories, to think that they are important. And people need to listen to the detail of the content, to the patterns, to the resonance with their own experiences

- Questioning rather than answering – people need to suspend their answer response which closes down dialogue, and instead engage in questioning, exploring, expanding, exploring issues more deeply
- "Re-experiencing the ordinary as extraordinary" (Shor, 1992: 122) occurs as people pose these questions and problematize social issues
- Collective action can then occur from a fully understood and explored issue with a range of potential solutions

In many respects, this story telling is a narrative research, and, beyond that, it is action research, and the individual narratives lead to collective understanding and collective or individual action. As McLaren (1995: 105) states, action research: "Aim[s] to construct counterstories that give shape and direction to the practice of hope and the struggle for an emancipatory politics of everyday life. It is a pedagogy that attempts to exorcise from the social body the invading pathologies of racism, sexism, and class privilege".

What does narrative theory offer the critical pedagogue? It is clear that narratives hold a great deal of potential for a critically pedagogical way of working in terms of using other people's narratives, understanding the group's past narrative and mapping a new future narrative.

You and the group may choose a published narrative or story and use it to compare to the group's experiences, and to unpack hidden messages. After reading a narrative you could ask if it resonates, and if so what the similarities are. You can explore strong liking and disliking of the narrative and where that came from. You can unpack the choices that the narrator made and the way that they present themselves.

You may be interested in why parables and fables came to be. You might become interested in the roles of women in stories and how that has changed over time. You might look at which narratives have become important and why that is. Whose narratives are published and whose never get seen? There are many fascinating questions to unravel.

The group may be interested in exploring their past by telling their stories and listening to one another (Ledwith, 2005), or mapping them visually on large pieces of wallpaper. The questions used to analyse the stories of other people can be applied to the group's own stories to reveal new understandings and meanings. This activity then leads naturally into creating and authoring a new future-facing narrative, enabling the group to chart what they want and how they will achieve it. Blogs and wikis offer exciting potential to publish narratives digitally enabling people to learn from and share personal stories globally.

In all narrative work, the critical pedagogue will be vigilant to the presence of prevalent discourses or hegemony. These are hidden messages buried in the events or the style of the story. One classic example of this is the hero's journey. Campbell (1990) identified the elements of a hero's journey as a grand narrative (large story) by which we all live our lives. The hero (usually male) is lost and alone, forsaken, overcomes great adversity and eventually triumphs through hardship and fortitude. The danger of us all adopting this narrative into our unconscious is that it can fuel us to work too hard, to be unforgiving of ourselves, and to expect success if we work hard enough. Awareness of such narratives can allow us to create alternatives – one of being peaceful and at one in the world, a narrative of connecting and aligning rather than combating and overcoming, a narrative of equality rather than of winning, a story where a woman as well as a man is valid. This early discussion of hidden messages leads nicely into the next section on media analysis.

Media critique

Media – be it a film, advert or news story, is designed to be engaging, so the media that you (or the group) have selected will be engaging and is a way into dialogue. Watching a film or looking at an image is potentially more inclusive than reading a book or newspaper as it overcomes the barrier of reading. In his book *Reading in the Dark* Golden (2001) advocates that film enables students to demonstrate critical thinking skills even if they have low reading skills in English classes. It is this critical thinking, rather than reading skill that is key to critical pedagogy.

The crucial idea to media critique, or critical media studies, is that you observe a media artefact and respond on two levels. The first level of analysis involves responding to the content of the piece, what was it about, what was the key message, etc. This can prompt agreement, disagreement, neutrality, different views, comparison to personal experience, discussion of alternatives and so on. This is rich analysis itself.

The second level of analysis is about the construction of the media artefact. Questions might include: who made the media artefact, and why they made it, what intentions the authors had, how they wanted the audience to react, who they intended to read it, what design choices were made and so on. Or in other words, how did the media author try to manipulate and control you? This surfaces understanding of hidden messages called discourse or hegemony in a fun and friendly manner!

Popular media provides a wealth of contemporary issues, societal norms, and a variety of perspectives. Further, it does this in a safe and engaging way. Here the group can talk about 'it' – the media artefact – rather than disclosing information about themselves. They can talk about the issue 'one step removed', rather than themselves personally. The may be a good way into open dialogue that is safe.

Dialogue about the artefact may well be ample learning itself. However, the group could also choose to respond. The group might want to write to the author expressing their views, they may wish to create an alternative artefact to publish in a counter-hegemonic way, or they may want to create an exposé, demonstrating the truth they have seen in the media artefact.

Social media makes responding to media artefacts so much easier. Many digital artefacts invite response in RSS feeds, and it is very simple to tweet and message reactions to what you have seen. Many young people have reacted strongly to inappropriate media artefacts, posted them online in wikis and blogs, and this has gone viral. This shows that the voices of the community can become as loud, if not louder than, those of the media thanks to social media – counter-hegemonic discourse is now ever present. An example of this people power is the reaction to Protein World's beach body ready poster for weight loss products featuring a thin model in a bikini. People defaced the posters, protesters posed in London in bikinis with 'this is a beach body' written on them, 60,000 people signed an online petition at Change.org and so on. Whilst the company did not remove the adverts or apologise, the adverts were banned from the London Tube. With social media literally at our fingertips, it is much simpler to create a message, movement and social change.

Creative arts – Theatre of the Oppressed

The Theatre of the Oppressed is a participative form of drama designed to be accessible. The process and content is designed for people who want to learn ways to fight back against the oppression they may experience in their everyday lives. Forum theatre and the Theatre of the Oppressed were designed by a Brazilian director and Workers' Party activist called Augusto Boal (1970). Unsurprisingly he was heavily influenced by Freire. The forum theatre is designed to problematise and increase conscientisation in just the same way as dialogue worked for Freire.

The actors in forum theatre typically begin with a dramatic situation from everyday life and try to find solutions from the audience. The audience can suggest what the actors might say and do, or even get up and replace them, acting themselves. This shifts the power of the theatre – usually shown to the audience, into something egalitarian and co-constructed. The audience get to rehearse and enact (literally) solutions to their everyday issues and see different perspectives and strategies tested out live. Boal called the audience "spect-actors" who "have the opportunity to both act and observe" and engage in "self-empowering processes of dialogue that help foster critical thinking". It is a "conscious intervention, as a rehearsal for social action rooted in a collective analysis of shared problems" (Brecht Forum Archive, 2016). Some of the tools to engage the audience are listed below:

Hot-Seating – The audience talk to the actors, who remain in character, and respond accordingly throughout the session, sometimes challenging the opinions put forward by the audience.

Re-direction – The audience examine an event or a character's behaviour/reactions and, in role as director, steer the scenario in a way they think might have different/better outcomes.

Think Bubbles – The facilitator asks what is going on in a character's head and the audience respond, filling in the imaginary thought bubble drawn above the character.

Hidden Voices – Audience members partner a character, and in the course of a scene's re-enactment, guide the professional actors in what they should say, or how they should react.

The sessions have a theatre facilitator who manages the dialogue and interaction between the audience and the actors. The aim is to explore as many solutions as possible, with the audience becoming empowered with their own sense of possibility. This scaffolds their ability to solve their own and wider social issues (Tait and Dunnett, 2012).

Running a forum theatre session need not be resource intensive. All you need is a couple of people to act out a situation. If your group is talking about a situation they were in and what they did, you can simply get up and act it out, saying 'did it look something like this?' From there it is a small step to ask for suggestions as to what else might be done. Initially the people might prefer to suggest alternatives rather than acting them out or you may find, as Boal did, that they get so frustrated that they simply jump up and take over.

Philosophy for children

Philosophy for children (P4C) creates communities of enquiry with school children. The approach was founded by Professor Matthew Lipman in 1972 and is grounded in the ideas of Vygotsky, Piaget, Dewey and the tradition of Socratic dialogue (SAPERE, 2016).

Typically participants sit in a circle and look at an image, object, or consider a phenomenon, such as bullying, as a stimulus. The children think of ideas for discussion (philosophical questions). These are written up on a board and the group collectively choose the question that most interests them to explore for the session. The discussion itself is open rather than structured, following the interests of the children, and conduct is governed by a contract set up and agreed by the group. An example of a philosophical question could be: 'is it ever OK to steal?' There is no judgement as to which is the 'best' question, only ever curiosity about which is the most interesting to the group to explore.

Some of the stated benefits of the P4C include:

- Learning to think before you speak
- Learning to give reasons for what you say
- Learning to value one another's contributions
- Learning that you do not have to be right
- Developing confidence to speak in a group
- Experiencing genuine enquiry
- Learning how to work collaboratively (Philosphy4Children, 2016).

Claims such as this are substantiated by an independent evaluation of P4C by the UK based Education Endowment Foundation (EEF, 2015). The randomised control trial involving over 3000 pupils found that:

the more disadvantaged pupils participating in the EEF trial saw their reading skills improve by four months, their maths results by three months and their writing ability by two months. Feedback from teachers throughout the trial suggests that Philosophy for Children had a beneficial impact on wider outcomes such as confidence, patience and self-esteem too (EEF, 2015).

Although established for children, the philosophical approach with structured stimulus and free flowing discussion can be powerful with groups of adult learners. As such the organisations SAPERE (2016) uses the 'C' in P4C to represent not only children, but also colleges and communities.

What does this approach offer the critical pedagogue? The structure of the sessions and use of stimulus materials may be helpful to you in creating a community of enquiry. The use of stimulus can usefully spark dialogue, teaching people how to question, as well as modelling critical pedagogical values such as collaborative working, mutual value and respect.

Reflective activity

Practice audit – complete the following table for your organisation, service or project.

Table 15.1 Analysis of personal use of critical pedagogical tools

	Consciously using	*Unconsciously using*	*Not using but could*	*Not using and unsuitable*
Third spaces				
Dialogue				
Narratives				
Media critique				
Creative arts				
Authentic learning				
P4C				
Mindfulness				

What steps do you think you might now take to develop more consciously critically pedagogical practice to support participants' wellbeing and social justice?

Evaluating wellbeing and social justice

You may be aiming to run a project for CYPF to develop awareness and critical consciousness, feel empowered and have choices, and take action. It is important to incorporate in the project design and development stage, how you evaluate to capture the process and any changes. This is an extension of your reflective practice, inherent within this approach, as it supports the better understanding, development and evidencing of your practice. Understanding, development and evidence are the three pillars of the Brathay Research Hub, where Kaz and Lucy developed much of their thinking around this book.

The word 'evaluation' can evoke the image of meaningless form filling! Most of us have been handed a questionnaire at the end of a training course to evaluate how well it worked. The problem with this kind of approach is that it is only benefitting the organisers. I usually don't get anything out of filling in one of those forms. At worst it is just a bureaucratic exercise, and at best it is for the organiser to say something about how well the course went so that s/he can run another.

We believe that evaluation should be for the benefit of all participants in all situations, but particularly when a project has a critically pedagogical approach. Imposing an end of project evaluation would irrevocably stamp your authority on what had been a democratic process. The way to overcome this issue is to establish participative action research (PAR) as a part of the project. PAR is a democratic form of research that seeks to achieve change. From that perspective it is entirely complementary to a critically pedagogical approach. PAR involves stakeholders in the design. The participants ask questions that are important to them in any given situation and choosing how they might collect data and analyse it. The practitioner can be the researcher and is part of the process rather than in control of the process – as in the critically pedagogical approach described throughout this text. PAR is also open to any data collection tools, there are no rules or restrictions to qualitative or quantitative, which enables it to be inclusive in style.

We have written elsewhere about the use of creative methods for evaluating practice (Stuart *et al.*, 2014). One of the key things is designing a theory of change to frame the project and evaluation. The essential components of this are:

- Context – needs, issues, assets
- Aim – the contribution of the project to the above context
- Outcomes – that breakdown the critical elements of the aim
- Process – the methods and activities you will use within a critical pedagogical approach to achieve the outcomes.

Most theories of change also include inputs (a numerical representation of the infrastructure put in place) and outputs (a numerical representation of the achievements – number of sessions delivered, attendance, facilitator hours).

The theory of change may be created with the participants, key stakeholders, or knowledgeable facilitators. This is a framework to guide this conversation, asking what's going on here, what do we want to learn or change, in what way, how shall we go about it, and, significantly – but usually forgotten – how shall we evaluate the process and impact?

Often evaluation is left to the end and is therefore seen as deciding which 'tool' to use. However, including it within the design stage makes us think about what we want to know and thus what questions we want to ask. This leads to the way we will find out and ensures we are not dictated to by a measurement or monitoring tool.

What this might mean for the critical pedagogue?

Our role is to problematise the evaluation process. This can include some of the following questions:

- What do you want to know and why?
- How would that help you?
- What would change look like, how would we know it had happened?
- What changes are important – how you think, feel, and act? Individual or collective?
- How could we collect that information?
- What would we do with the information? Who would be involved in that?
- Who might be interested in what we find out and why?

Further reading

Critical Pedagogical Teaching Ideas in The Barefoot Guides: http://www.barefoot guide.org/

The Philosophy for Children Resource Database: http://www.sapere.org.uk/Default.aspx? tabid=289

Critical pedagogical lesson plans available here: http://www.freireproject.org/resources/ in-the-classroom/lesson-plans/

The International Journal of Critical Pedagogy: http://libjournal.uncg.edu/ijcp

Resources for dialogue: http://elac.ex.ac.uk/dialogiceducation/page.php?id=119

Theatre of the Oppressed toolkit: https://www.salto-youth.net/tools/toolbox/tool/theatre-of-the-oppressed-resource-manual.1475/

Authentic Learning for Literacy Toolkit: http://www.ncsall.net/fileadmin/resources/teach/ jacobson.pdf

Storytelling resources: http://www.timsheppard.co.uk/story/tellinglinks.html

Digital storytelling resources: http://www.techsoup.org/community/community-initiatives/ storymakers-resources

Sources of free, licence free, movie clips: http://www.movieclips.com/

Duncan-Andrade, J. M., and Morrell, E. (2008). *The Art of Critical Pedagogy: Possibilities for Moving from Theory to Practice in Urban Schools.* New York: Peter Lang Publishing.

Horsley, K. and necf (2016). *The Evaluator's Cookbook.* Accessed on 4/9/16 at: http:// www.bath.ac.uk/marketing/public-engagement/assets/the_evaluators_cookbook_ participatory_evaluation_exercises_for_young_people.pdf

References

Bettelheim, B. (1976). *The Uses of Enchantment: The Meaning and Importance of Fairy Tales.* New York: Knopf.

Boal, A. (1970). *Theatre of the Oppressed.* New York: Routledge.

Brecht Forum Archive (2016). *Augusto Boal and the Theatre of the Oppressed.* Accessed on 26. 8. 16 at: https://brechtforum.org/abouttop

Campbell, J. (1968). *The Hero with a Thousand Faces.* New York: Meridian Books.

Campbell, J. (1990). *The Hero's Journey.* Novato, CA: New World Library.

Chisholm, L. (2000). *Charting a Hero's Journey.* New York: The International Partnership for Service-Learning.

Clandinin, C., and Connelly, F. (1994). *Narrative Inquiry.* San Francisco: Jossey-Bass.

Clandinin, D., and Connelly, F. (2000). *Narrative Inquiry.* San Francisco: Jossey-Bass.

Denning, S. (2005). *The Leaders Guide to Storytelling.* San Francisco: Jossey-Bass.

Education Endowment Foundation (EEF) (2015). *Philosophy for Children.* Accessed on 25. 8. 16 at: https://educationendowmentfoundation.org.uk/evaluation/projects/philosophy-for-children

educNET (2016). *Dialogic Teaching and Learning.* Accessed on 26. 8. 16 at: https://www.educ.cam.ac.uk/research/projects/camtalk/dialogic/

Freire, P. (1970). *Pedagogy of the Oppressed.* New York: Seabury.

Freire, P. (1973). *Education for a Critical Consciousness.* New York: Seabury Press.

Golden, J. (2001). *Reading in the Dark: Using Film as a Tool in the English Classroom.* New York: National Council of Teachers.

Gutierrez, K. (2008). 'Developing a Sociocritical Literacy in the Third Space', *Reading Research Quarterly*, 43(2), 148–164.

Hill Collins, P. (1990). *Black Feminist Thought: Knowledge, Consciousness and the Politics of Empowerment.* Boston: Unwin Hyman.

Kouzes, J., and Posner, B. (2003). *Encouraging The Heart: A Leader's Guide to Rewarding and Recognizing Others.* San Francisco: Jossey-Bass.

Ledwith, M. (2005). *Community Development: A Critical Approach.* London: Polity Presss.

Ledwith, M. (2016). *Community Development in Action. Putting Freire into Practice.* Bristol: Policy Press.

McLaren, P. (1995). *Critical Pedagogy and Predatory Culture: Oppositional Politics in a Postmodern Era.* London: Routledge.

Moje, E. B., Ciechanowski, K. M., Kramer, K., Ellis, L., Carillo, R., and Collazo, T. (2004). 'Working Toward Third Space in Content Area Literacy. An Examination of Everyday Funds of Knowledge and Discourse', *Reading Research Quarterly*, 39, 38–70.

Morgan, A. (2000). *What is Narrative Therapy?* Adelaide: Dulwich Centre Publications.

Pahl, K. and Kelly, S. (2005). 'Family Literacy as a Third Space Between Home and School: Some Case Studies of Practice', *Literacy*, 39: 91–96.

Philosophy4Children (2016). 'What is Philosophy for Children?' Accessed on 25. 8. 16 at: http://www.philosophy4children.co.uk/home/p4c/

Parkin, M. (2001). *Tales for Trainers.* London: Kogan Page.

Ryan, G. (2016). 'Learn About the Seven Skills of Dialogue'. Accessed on 25. 8. 16 at: http://planforpersonalsuccess.com/learn-about-the-seven-skills-of-dialogue/

Saleha Gandana, I. (2008). 'Exploring Third Spaces: Negotiating Identities and Cultural Differences', *The International Journal of Diversity in Organisations, Communities and Nations*, 7(6), 143–150.

SAPERE (2016). 'What is P4C?' Accessed on 24. 8. 16 at: http://www.sapere.org.uk/default.aspx?tabid=162

Shor, I. (1992). *Empowering Education: Critical Teaching for Social Change*. Chicago: University of Chicago Press.

Souto-Manning, M. (2009). *Freire, Teaching, and Learning: Culture Circles across Contexts*. New York: Peter Lang.

Stuart, K., Maynard, L., and Rouncefield, C. (2014). *Evaluating Projects with Young People: Creative Research Methods*. London: Sage.

Tait, J., and Dunnett, R. (2012). *Introducing Forum Theatre*. Ireland: National Association of Youth Drama.

Thomas, T., and Killick, S. (2007). *Telling Tales, Storytelling as Emotional Literacy*. Blackburn: Educational Printing Services.

White, M. (2007). *Maps of Narrative Practice*. New York: Norton.

Vogler, C. (2007). *The Writer's Journey: Mythic Structure for Storytellers and Screenwriters*. Studio City, CA: Michael Wiese Productions.

Walther, S., and Carey, M. (2009). 'Narrative Therapy, Difference and Possibility: Inviting New Becomings', *Context*, October, 2007.

Conclusion

Throughout the book we have established that wellbeing is feeling good and functioning well, and that it is inextricably linked to social justice, which we define as equality, equity and the ability to use capabilities to function freely in the world. This is personal, social and political. We argue that the process of empowerment enables people to use their agency (comprised of awareness, choices and actions) to minimise the impact of constraining structures, and to lever the possibility of enabling structures. Empowerment to support the state of agency is critically important in enabling people to create their own wellbeing and social justice. We summarised this conceptual framework in the model in chapter 7, shown again below.

We have presented the breadth and complexity of this by gradually building up our framework for practice throughout the chapters. This is exemplified in the case studies, as they are analysed inwards through the concentric circles of the model, ascertaining what 'was' before the project or service, and then working outwards through the concentric circles of the model to understand what changes happened as a result of the critical pedagogical work.

We have positioned critical pedagogy as a practice approach that is at the heart of the conceptual framework. It is by working with people in a critically pedagogical way that we can support empowerment and agency. A critically pedagogical approach directly supports wellbeing and social justice as they are implicit aims of the approach and are supported secondarily as a result of enhanced empowerment and agency. It is as if working in a critically pedagogical way creates a virtual spiral of positive outcomes.

The projects have all been structured to develop critical consciousness or awareness, to give the participants real and meaningful choices, and to support them to an agentic state. The process of empowerment is evident in them all – realising, wanting, committing and development of skills are apparent. Some of the CYPF and practitioners recycle and need additional support, and we now understand this to be a positive experience.

Therefore, we have several key messages for practice: you cannot do empowerment to CYPF; our work supports them to become empowered. Equally, you cannot do wellbeing and social justice to CYPF; our work supports them to grow their own wellbeing and develop social justice for themselves

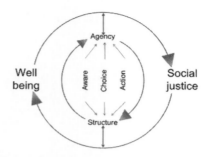

Figure C.1 The Wellbeing and Social Justice Model

and others – families, communities, projects, organisations. This is a process of sustainable change because it is intrinsically driven and thus owned, developed and nurtured by CYPF.

Of course, as practitioners we are not redundant in this. We have power, but so do CYPF and this is always visible and available to work with. We have knowledge, but so do CYPF and so our work is experiential. Our role is as facilitator of this process, both catalytic and knowledgeable of what could be. This model therefore is a framework to support and guide practice. It can help design, deliver and evaluate practice. It provides an underpinning to support work that may need to spend an awful lot of time at the awareness phase and that this is a vital grounding.

The final chapter identifying critical pedagogical practices highlights ways in which we can practically support wellbeing and social justice. The example practices are not an exhaustive list, they are only the tip of the iceberg, but they detail what it was that enabled wellbeing outcomes to be achieved in the case studies.

We hope that you have gained the sense that it is not so much what you do, but how you do it that matters. All of your choices as a practitioner are important, you therefore need to apply critical pedagogical approach to your own work, questioning what you are doing and why.

We hope that some of the vague language used has been grounded in concrete terms in this book. Wellbeing and social justice are the overall **aims** of our work. The **process** of empowerment supports people to arrive at a state of enhanced agency. Agency is comprised of awareness, choices and actions, and is what we all use to navigate the structures that surround us. Critical pedagogy is the **approach** framing what we do on the ground. We have grounded these abstract terms in very real examples of practice and hope that these have also illuminated them as multi-disciplinary, intergenerational, and equally applicable to practitioners as to CYPF.

Maxine Greene suggests that;

> We need to teach in such a way as to arouse passion now and then; we need a new camaraderie, a new en masse. These are dark and shadowed

times, and we need to live in them, standing before one another, open to the world (2009: 96).

We hope that this book will create this camaraderie and en masse. We have attempted to raise awareness of what critical pedagogy is theoretically and practically and why it is important for global wellbeing and social justice. We hope that the case studies and examples of key practices will enable you to choose to work in a critically pedagogical way. We now hand over to you, to take action, to go out into the dark and shadowed times to create some light.

References

Greene, M. (2009). "In Search of a Critical Pedagogy', in Darder, A., Baltodano, M., and Torres, R. (eds), *The Critical Pedagogy Reader* (2nd edn). New York: Routledge.

Index

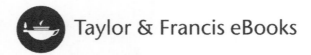

Taylor & Francis eBooks

Helping you to choose the right eBooks for your Library

Add Routledge titles to your library's digital collection today. Taylor and Francis ebooks contains over 50,000 titles in the Humanities, Social Sciences, Behavioural Sciences, Built Environment and Law.

Choose from a range of subject packages or create your own!

Benefits for you

>> Free MARC records
>> COUNTER-compliant usage statistics
>> Flexible purchase and pricing options
>> All titles DRM-free.

Benefits for your user

>> Off-site, anytime access via Athens or referring URL
>> Print or copy pages or chapters
>> Full content search
>> Bookmark, highlight and annotate text
>> Access to thousands of pages of quality research at the click of a button.

REQUEST YOUR **FREE** INSTITUTIONAL TRIAL TODAY | **Free Trials Available** We offer free trials to qualifying academic, corporate and government customers.

eCollections – Choose from over 30 subject eCollections, including:

Archaeology	Language Learning
Architecture	Law
Asian Studies	Literature
Business & Management	Media & Communication
Classical Studies	Middle East Studies
Construction	Music
Creative & Media Arts	Philosophy
Criminology & Criminal Justice	Planning
Economics	Politics
Education	Psychology & Mental Health
Energy	Religion
Engineering	Security
English Language & Linguistics	Social Work
Environment & Sustainability	Sociology
Geography	Sport
Health Studies	Theatre & Performance
History	Tourism, Hospitality & Events

For more information, pricing enquiries or to order a free trial, please contact your local sales team:
www.tandfebooks.com/page/sales

 Routledge Taylor & Francis Group | The home of Routledge books | **www.tandfebooks.com**